**Where Did All the Fat Go?
The WOW! ℞**

LOSE FAT—GAIN MUSCLE!

Where Did All the Fat Go?

The WOW! ℞

ROB HUIZENGA, M.D.

From the Doctor Behind the Hit NBC-TV Show,

The Biggest Loser

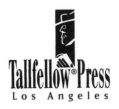

Tallfellow®Press
Los Angeles

Exercise photos by Muriel Mutzel
Contestant graduation photos by Harry Haese
Contestant group photos by Tiare White
Cover/jacket design by Pamela Pollock

Published by
Tallfellow® Press, Inc.
1180 S. Beverly Drive
Los Angeles, California 90035
www.Tallfellow.com

ISBN: 978-1-931290-57-9

Printed in the United States of America.

10 9 8 7 6 5 4 3 2 1

Disclaimer

All weight-loss programs have risks. This dramatic fat-loss, health enhancement program is rigorous. Therefore, it is necessary for you to be pre-screened by your physician to determine whether your current physical condition is adequate to permit you to embark on this program, which includes vigorous exercise. After starting this program, proper screening and monitoring by your physician is required to ensure that your ongoing health condition permits you to continue. Although the WOW! ℞ has been proven to be safe and tolerable, even for morbidly obese individuals, it is not the intent of the author to directly or indirectly diagnose, dispense medical advice, or prescribe the use of this program as a form of treatment for medical problems. If you use the information contained in this book without the approval of your physician, the publisher and author assume no responsibility for your actions.

This exercise and fat-loss plan is not appropriate for pregnant women. Women have become pregnant while following the WOW! ℞—weight loss enhances fertility; weight loss during pregnancy could, in fact, be detrimental to the health and safety of both mother and child!

This book is dedicated:

*to the hundreds of Biggest Loser participants, thanks for
the inspiration and the all-access pass to the overweight world.*

*to Wanda, thanks for the all-access pass to love
(and for monitoring my chocolate intake).*

*to the memory of my mom, thanks for the all-access
pass to life (and for introducing me to chocolate!).*

People try to lose weight to get healthy.

They've got it inside out and backward—

You need to lose fat, not "weight,"

And you've got to get healthy in order to lose fat.

Dr. Rob Huizenga

Contents

Acknowledgments

My sincerest thanks to Larry Sloan and Claudia Sloan of Tallfellow Press for shepherding this book from start to finish, to Linda Laucella for her exceptional editing and organizational skills, Jen Kerns for "insider" weight-loss knowledge, Dr. Michael Dansinger, Dr. Alexa Altman, Dr. Michael Brousseau, Meg Werner Moreta RD, Jim Matthie, Lisa Singer, Pete Koch, Rena Copperman, Bob Tinnon, Michael Sund, Janis Uhley, Janna Wong Healy, Monica Ek, the entire staff of *The Biggest Loser*, and my dad, Dr. John R. Huizenga, for being a role-model scientist.

Prologue

Where Did All the Fat Go?

E-mail flagged urgent:

Dear Dr. Huizenga,
I just weighed myself. . .and that scale was undoubtedly at 177!!! I mean, it may be 178 later as it fluctuates throughout the day, but this morning, there was no ambiguity. . . . The scale told me plain as day that I've lost 100 pounds!!!!!!!!!!!!!!

I absolutely got tears in my eyes. . . . I just cannot believe it! When I went to the open *Biggest Loser* audition in Boston, I wrote on the application that I wanted to lose 100 pounds. . .but at the time that seemed impossible, especially for a nonathletic woman! I just chose an arbitrary number that I thought sounded big enough to get me on the show! And then of course when I wasn't selected for the show, I figured it was absolutely impossible!!!!!!!!!!!!!

Now two more pounds and I will be at my weight from when I was fifteen. I have not weighed what I weigh this minute in twelve years! I cannot believe this!!! Where did all the fat go??????

Congratulations! We're early in the fifth month, and already—totally on your own at home—you're a triple-digit fat loser!!! (P.S. I'm thinking the last pound of fat loss was you hitting that exclamation key!!) I love your "where-did-all-the-fat-go" question! You probably intended it as a rhetorical figure of speech, but as you can well imagine, I'm all worked up over the scientific and health implications. . . .
Dr. H.

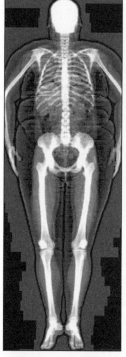
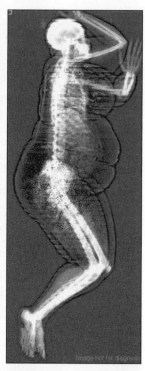

These eye-opening day one front and side view iDEXA scans reveal a "normal body" (muscles and organs gray) buried beneath the layers of fat (black).

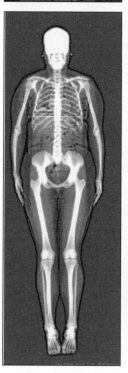
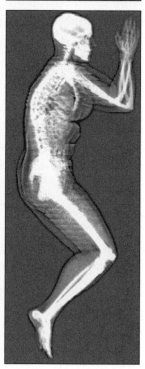

After 100 pounds of fat loss (and slight muscle gain) on the WOW! Rx, the "normal body" is liberated!

Introduction

Lose Fat, Not "Weight" with The WOW! ℞ to Get Back into Your "Thin" Clothes... and Your Life

Are you overweight or obese? Do you have visible fat rolls? Are you greater than 15 to 20 pounds heavier than your weight at age 21? Have you gone on "health" kicks and tried to lose weight with Atkins, Ornish, Weight Watchers, the Zone, or any other trendy diet program? Have you—like the subjects in two just-published medical studies—lost only 5 to 10 pounds after months, or even a year, of dieting? Worse yet, has the weight boomeranged back within a few years? Contemplating throwing out all your "thin" clothes? Or have you been "chubby" since childhood, and never owned "thin" clothes at all? Convinced you'll be fat your whole life because there's something wrong with your metabolism? Or are you now so determined to get "healthy" that you're considering drastic measures... miracle wraps... never-tested Internet-touted weight-loss potions... off-label prescription drugs... or even stomach bypass surgery?

STOP! Stop trying to lose weight to get healthy. You've got it inside out and backward—you need to lose fat, not "weight," and you've got to get healthy in order to lose fat.

The WOW! ℞ is a scientific fat-loss prescription for overweight, obese, and morbidly obese people who are truly serious about losing toxic excess fat without sacrificing water, muscle, and bone. The WOW! ℞ gets you fit, thereby enabling you to sensibly lose "big" amounts of fat—and keep it off.

Why is The WOW! ℞ program different from every other available diet program?

- The WOW! ℞ works with—not counter to—your innate survival instincts.

- The WOW! ℞ can result in dramatic fat loss over six months—averaging two to 10 times more than other home-based programs—based on medical studies of 172 *The Biggest Loser* contestants (including contestants who participated on their own at home, without the help of trainers).
- The WOW! ℞ can result in fat loss equal to the most aggressive gastric bypass weight-loss surgery. In a number of cases, morbidly obese individuals were able to get down to their ideal **With-Out-Waist** fat weight (**WOW!** weight) in just six months!
- The rapid visible weight loss associated with The WOW! ℞ serves as an important motivator; similarly, the closer you get to your WOW! weight—a truly life-altering event—the greater your incentive to keep it all off.
- By following The WOW! ℞, you lose, essentially, all fat! By preserving calorie-hungry lean tissue, The WOW! ℞ sets you up for long-term success; maintaining or in many cases gaining muscle through exercise helps keep your metabolic rate as high as possible which is critical for preventing weight regain. I have followed the weight-loss maintenance of all participants, and the results after one to two years are substantially better than any other available diet.
- The WOW! ℞ reliably reduces heartburn, asthma, snoring, high cholesterol, high blood pressure, and diabetes. Astonishingly, a high percentage of smokers have quit while simultaneously losing significant amounts of fat.
- The WOW! ℞ addresses psychological impediments to weight loss. It improves energy, happiness, and overall quality of life. In fact, most successful participants had no idea just how lethargic and depressed they were feeling until after their WOW! ℞ "transformations."
- The WOW! ℞ corrects difficult-to-detect but damaging inflammation and pre-diabetes conditions that can signal a shortened life span of up to 20 years in seriously obese young persons.

- All weight-loss diets have risks. When candidates are properly screened and monitored by their physicians, The WOW! ℞ has been proven to be safe and tolerable, even for morbidly obese individuals.
- The WOW! ℞ is the road map to a total body transformation, but does require a commitment. You must set aside the appropriate time—for some people as much as two hours a day to exercise—an extra hour to shop, plan, and prepare meals, and you must be motivated. You must embrace vitality and quality of life over lethargy and early death.

Three years ago, before I witnessed doctors, lawyers, working and stay-at-home moms (with no help!), cops, firefighters, pilots, businessmen and women, teachers, drivers, realtors. . . you name it. . . finding the time to work out twice a day, and getting hooked on the exercise "high," I would have dismissed The WOW! ℞ as laughingly impractical. But over the last four years, I've seen it work time and time again with my own eyes. It is absolutely do-able. Every contestant that returned for the finale of *The Biggest Loser* television show lost significant amounts of fat; the majority lost massive amounts of fat. Best of all, early indications after one to two years of follow-up are that they're also keeping the fat off!

——— ———

Are you overweight, obese, or morbidly obese? Are you seriously out of shape? Give your body the attention it deserves; embrace The WOW! ℞—then get back into your "thin" clothes. . . and your life!

SECTION ONE

GET WITH THE PROGRAM

The ABCs of the R$_x$

Chapter One

The Biggest Loser: The Bumpy Road to Malibu

August 10, 2004. It was the first week of the very first The Biggest Loser *television show. The contestants' weight was dropping off in 10-, 15-, even 20-plus pound chunks. It was like a scene out of* Honey, I Shrunk the Kids! *They were growing thinner, literally, on a day-to-day basis, in front of my eyes. Their joints were achy, their muscles sore, a few had cramps, but at 8 o'clock in the morning, every one of these former couch potatoes was ready to exercise again. No one was hungry; you could have boarded them in a gingerbread house or made it rain fresh-baked donuts, and no one would have taken a bite.*

I was scared. During my 25-year medical career, I'd never seen, heard, or read about anything quite like this.

I didn't start out as a weight-loss doctor, as such; I specialize in internal medicine and sports medicine. I never dreamed that one day I'd find myself documenting a natural weight-loss treatment plan that was as potent as gastric bypass surgery—with far fewer complications—but, in retrospect, I realize that I've been in training for this discovery my entire life.

Practically my first recollection is of my chubby mom, God rest her soul, rummaging through family albums, proudly pointing to a bathing-suit photo of her taken on a Lake Michigan sand dune—"After four kids, mind you," she'd shamelessly assert—where she had Hollywood legs and nary a drop of waist fat. But while I grew up thin—playing round-the-clock sports—she yo-yoed from overweight to obese, despite an annoying array of deprivation diets. After our so-called "health-conscious" double-dinner servings of bread, meat, potatoes, and vegetables— topped with volumes of butter, gravy, sour cream, and dessert fruit with thick cream (Mom was a nurse and made a point of insisting we get all the food groups)—the family banter would eventually drift to her next empty diet vow or the latest worthless waist-reduction remedy.

Then, at the age of 13, it was suddenly my turn to cut weight. I was a skinny 115-pound freshman, so why on earth would I need to lose weight? Well, a double disaster hit, leaving me no other choice. One, I stopped growing at 5′ 4″ (5′ 5″ with the folded newspaper I inserted in my penny loafers) and two, we moved to a district with 5,000-plus kids in my high school (i.e., the sports teams were tough to make). My parents said I was too small for football and refused to sign the medical release, so I practiced nonstop for basketball, my best sport. Unfortunately, at the last cut for the freshman basketball team, a bunch of us were standing outside the boys' gym at 2:30 in the afternoon when the coach tacked up the handwritten list of those who made the team. I can still see it: My name was not there. I plummeted through embarrassment to depression, then utter humiliation. I'd always been the star player. I couldn't go home, much less face my friends. Then, noticing the wrestling room, I flashed on the solution. How hard could wrestling be? How many athletic kids of my height could there be? Too hard and too many, it turned out. The freshman team had 12 members in the 112-pound weight class, and one of them, Cory (I found out later that he was the coach's son), kicked the living crap out of me in practice. It was obvious that my only hope would be the 103-pound weight class with only eight members on the challenge board.

I came home, told my mom to buy a case of diet cola, and basically stopped eating. As I watched my puny arm muscles fade to nothing, I knew starvation was stupid, but when I beat the other boys for the 103-pound roster spot—and had my first drink of water in a day—it suddenly seemed very worthwhile.

To stay weight competitive on the squad, I lost, then gained, 10 to 20 pounds a week—week after week. A few years into my high school sports career, I'd already lost (and gained) more pounds than any contestant on *The Biggest Loser*. I'd become a world-class yo-yo dieter. When I went on to college, the pressure to cut weight to remain competitive as a wrestler was even more extreme. A few days before a weigh-in, the real fight would begin, with willpower-battling, raging appetite. I was non-stop hungry. While doing homework in the kitchen, I'd open the fridge door maybe a hundred times a day, staring blankly at the vegetables and diet cola bottles I was rationing. Each night I tossed and turned to food-themed dreams. Pre-weigh-in days were a disaster. Walking to class with muscles stripped of glycogen, I felt like Superman carrying Kryptonite books. Standing up after class? Forget it! A dehydration faint was inevitable unless I got up in slow motion.

But I learned a lot! I was cutting less weight than many of my team-mates, so just hanging out in the training room was like a fellowship at an unlicensed weight-loss clinic. I witnessed every ugly corner-cutting trick: no-carb, no-fat, or no-calorie diets; dehydration; diuretics; stimulants; laxatives; enemas and even helium enemas (teaching wrestlers the weight of inert gases in sophomore chemistry can be hazardous to their health); nonstop exercise; exercising in plastic sweats; exercising in plastic sweats in saunas; spitting; induced vomiting; scale tampering—you name it. Before long—even before I discovered that my mom's perfect swimsuit picture had been courtesy of prescription amphetamines—I learned all about "rebound," with wrestling buddies withdrawing from stimulants, persistently vomiting immediately after meals, and bingeing like there was no tomorrow—oh, yes, losing weight the wrong way can develop into anorexia and/or uncontrollable bingeing—some blimping up as much as 50 pounds in just a few weeks!

I knew weight loss was stupid, but when I returned to Ann Arbor from the national tournament, having just finished my college-wrestling career as an NCAA All-American, it all seemed very worthwhile. Then, later that night, the sinister side of messing with Mother Nature's appetite controls hit home. I realized I had a problem that I could not control. I couldn't stop eating. Despite having eaten dinner earlier, the minute I got to my cramped attic apartment, I cooked a chicken and mixed up a whole box of the tapioca pudding I'd dreamed about the week before. I multiplied the ingredients by 16, bringing a gallon of milk to a slow boil, and then devoured it all in a single sitting—despite the onset of searing pains halfway through. The incessant dieting had scrambled the hunger wiring in my brain, but I naively assumed that the brain-stomach disconnect was as short-term and reversible as my college parka. Again, I was dead wrong.

During my first weekend at medical school, a parallel concern surfaced, preposterous as it now sounds: Were the one to two hours of exercise I was doing daily actually bad for me? I know, it sounds crazy, but 25 years ago it was widely believed by the medical community (and general public) that exercise was actually bad for you! So now, not only was I struggling with binge eating, I was also about to be told that exercise was detrimental to my health. After getting caught in a scrum (that's a clutch of rugby guys fighting for a leather ball) and separating my right shoulder, I stiffly sat, with my shoulder braced to my waist, in the regal quadrangle office of my academic advisor, a world-renowned pathologist, as he lectured me: "You shouldn't have been playing rugby on Harvard Medical School's time. You'll soon learn that extreme exertion is bad for the heart, and furthermore, sports detract from the single-minded focus a Harvard doctor must possess."

While I eyed the exit door, he conveyed his own workout philosophy with a sly grin, "When I go to the track, it's to bet on horses."

I immediately dismissed my advisor's "academic-focus" warning because I'd gotten my best grades while playing intercollegiate sports. If I weren't actively training, my concentration ebbed, I'd fade out in class and spend more of my free time drinking cheap pink Chablis, crashing sorority mixers, and patronizing—you guessed it—all-you-can-eat-buffets. When I wasn't fit, I simply didn't feel right. But maybe exercise was a bad addiction? As I furiously pedaled along the Charles River (biking was the only exercise my aching shoulder could handle), I began to worry. Was exercise shortening my life? Common sense told me no, and at 22 years of age, I was skeptical of anyone over 30, no matter the size of their office or number of framed Ivy League diplomas on their walls.

Four years later, the worry returned with a vengeance. I'd barely unpacked my bags for an internship at Cedars-Sinai Medical Center in Los Angeles—one of the country's top heart hospitals—when I admitted a man who'd suffered a heart attack after his morning jog. The chief of cardiology dissected the case on ward rounds, reiterating the folly of vigorous activity and his belief that, at best, even mild exercise was of no benefit. And then, like the cavalry riding to the rescue, a landmark study appeared in 1984, proving these doctors dead wrong (whew!). The *Cliffs-Notes* version: In well-conditioned individuals, the risk of death subtly increased during vigorous exercise; however, the risk of death was tremendously lower for the remaining 23 hours of the day. Net effect? Exercise is a lifesaver—the more, the better. My mentors failed to recognize the single most powerful feel-good, look-good, be-healthy, and live-long potion known to man (and woman). Everybody makes mistakes, but before this, I never thought a renowned cardiology department chief (who, incidentally, had a pot belly, was sedentary, and suffered a stroke in his 60s) or an Ivy League M.D.–Ph.D. type (also had a pot belly, was sedentary, and died in his 60s) could be so dead wrong.

Oddly enough, one of my first jobs as a full-fledged doctor was to prevent weight loss. NFL players need equal parts bulk and quickness to dominate an opponent, but as the Los Angeles Raiders' team physician, I saw the weight of our big linemen essentially evaporate during intense two-a-day pre-season practices. I struggled to keep their weight on with team buffets supplemented with round-the-clock room service pizzas and Häagen-Dazs shakes, anything to prevent them from resorting to the shadowy world of anabolic steroids and growth hormones for a bigger body.

In my other life as a private-practice internist, I treated tons of overweight patients engaged in a battle to prevent weight gain or an all-out war to permanently lose weight. Before long I recognized—in between the jumble of low-fat, low-carb, low-calorie food versus liquid-only diets—that the patients who were successful at losing fat and keeping it off were exercisers! Many ate large quantities of food (like me), but regularly worked it off (like me). I preached from my soapbox, telling anyone within earshot that "dumbed-down" exercise (a 30-minute walk three to four times a week) slightly improves health, but is worthless for weight loss. I tried my hardest to refute my patients' "I don't have time" lie and their "I can't eat healthy" hoax, begging them to step up their exercise routines. But I could see my patients' eyes glazing over—by the time I ticked off the amazingly low obesity rates in the Amish community, where they eat lots of high-fat foods but do six or more hours of daily manual labor. . . by the time I mentioned "portion control". . . loud snoring echoed throughout my office. Something was missing from my spiel!

So when a team of young TV turks from Universal—not the theme park, but the real studio, they assured me—asked for my help on an as-yet-untitled weight-loss reality show, I was intrigued. In contrast to the nip-tuck reality shows—*Extreme Makeover, The Swan,* and *Dr. 90210*—the idea for this show was low tech and deceptively simple: follow a group of obese contestants as they exercise and diet, and hopefully end up changing their appearances and their lives. Considering the plethora of plastic surgery-themed shows on prime time, this all-natural transformation concept was a breath of fresh air. NBC loved the idea; the timing was right; the spin-off possibilities were unlimited. Just one pesky detail remained.

"Doc, what's the most weight someone could safely lose in 10 weeks?"

They had already told me that giving the contestants more time to lose weight was not an option. The network would be paying top dollar to house their 12 weight-losing contestants and shoot the show in just 10 weeks, translating into a series of eight televised shows. Furthermore, most previous reality shows were filmed over shorter periods of time and were considerably cheaper to produce.

"Through aggressive dieting alone, you can expect at most a fraction over 1 percent weight loss per week during the first month or two—30 pounds over 10 weeks for a 300-pounder—a bit less with a low-fat plan because there's less water loss," I answered. "But no one has ever tacked on two-a-day exercise," I said as I flashed back to professional football summer camp. "Mix in vigorous exercise with intense interval training and you might see something special. Maybe double the standard weight loss!"

"If it's never been studied, how can you be sure?" they asked.

I had a quick answer: "When I was with the Raiders, I was supposed to keep the 300-pound nose tackles at 300 pounds. But when they were exerting strenuously four hours a day, despite practically holding their heads in a feeding trough the rest of the day, they dropped weight. When you work out that hard, fat just disappears."

"Well, how much weight loss? This is TV, Doc. For this show to sail, we've got to actually see a difference."

For the first time I saw what was at stake. The brash TV producers, Mark Koops and JD Roth, under the gleaming 30-year-old eyes of wunderkind Ben Silverman, were investing millions of dollars in an experiment, variations of which the medical community had tried countless times before, with uniformly underwhelming results.

I mumbled through a 10-second guesstimate: A 300-pounder could safely lower food intake by 1,000 calories a day (that's 7,000 calories per week), 3,500 calories equal 1 pound of fat, so 7,000 calories amount to a loss of 2 pounds of fat per week. Adding two-a-day workouts could theoretically triple that fat loss: 2,000 calories burned every day during three snappy exercise hours equal 14,000 calories burned, or up to 4 extra pounds of fat lost per week. I threw out a number, "Your winners could show 60 pounds of fat loss in 10 weeks. Now, if they stick to a low-carb diet—which will hurt their ability to exercise, and would be counterproductive in the long term—then tack on another 10 to 20 pounds of water and muscle loss. The TV cameras might spot facial changes at 10 pounds of fat loss. At 60 pounds—half a normal-sized adult—the difference will jump off the airwaves and slap the home audience in the face."

During a subsequent conversation, I was conferenced in with skeptical network execs. Again I blithely tossed out my optimistic 10-week best-case estimate for a flabby 300- or 400-pound contestant, "60 to 70 pounds lost."

"Our doctors here in New York quoted from medical journals citing that 3 pounds per week is the most they'll lose; 25 to 30 pounds max over 10 weeks!" one insistent female exec retorted.

Imagine you're an established doctor, Clinical Associate Professor of Medicine at UCLA, a past president of the NFL Physicians Society—could anything be more embarrassing than getting sandbagged by a 20-something reality TV vice president spouting medical lingo and posturing like an Ivy League medical subspecialist? Especially when she's correct! No outpatient food-based diet study had ever documented more than a 30-pound weight loss over this short of a time span. However, I was aware of in-hospital starvation studies (zero-caloric intakes) with 300-plus-pound patients dropping up to 18 pounds per week—of course only a third of that initial weight drop was fat (the rest was water and lean tissue/muscle loss)—and after several weeks, the starvation weight loss stabilized to 7 pounds per week, with fat accounting for about 60 to 70 percent of that loss.

The network brass felt this show, now tentatively called *The Biggest Loser*, could be a hit if my calculations were correct. Then reality really hit me. My diet plan differed radically from all prior obesity studies because none had ever followed participants who achieved weight loss by combining vigorous exercise with a moderate-calorie diet of healthful food. If I was wrong, and the contestants on this new reality show were unable to drop dramatic amounts of fat, "I told you so" would be splashed across millions of TV screens. Scarier still, as I ran the numbers through my head for the umpteenth time, I realized I was recommending fewer calories than starvation! Sure, a 300-pound *Biggest Loser* contestant would eat five meals equaling up to 1,800 calories per day, but compared to someone sitting in a hospital ward in a starvation study, he or she would burn 2,000 or even 3,000 calories per day during the twice-daily exercise sessions. So, net, they'd "take in" less than zero calories!

"Six pounds is a lot to lose in one week," the TV exec repeated, rousing me from my worst-case scenario thoughts.

"I used to lose 12 pounds in a single wrestling workout!" I quickly interjected. "I've seen a 300-pound lineman lose 26 pounds in one game!"

I tried to distract her with meaningless water-loss stories until I could better research the advisability of my less-than-zero approach.

FAST FORWARD: MALIBU, CALIFORNIA
INTERIOR: *THE BIGGEST LOSER* RANCH

I was too nervous to sleep the night before I met the contestants on the inaugural *The Biggest Loser* television show. No one had ever before dared to try an approach like this, and I was scared that it would fail. Would a weight-loss method conceived from observations on elite professional athletes and brought to fruition through the out-of-the-box thinking of a bunch of television executives actually work with morbidly obese desk jockeys? Would it work with sedentary individuals who'd collectively lost and regained hundreds of pounds on every conceivable commercial diet plan? Would it work with contestants who had serious diseases—asthma, hypertension, diabetes, acid reflux, and sleep apnea—lurking under every belly roll?

Could couch potatoes survive three to four hours of exercise per day? No matter how motivated the mind, would the body respond? Would injuries sideline the entire lot? Even more importantly, could they be reprogrammed to exercise and eat with discipline, even after the show ended?

The weight-loss program worked. The obese and morbidly obese couch-potato contestants quickly ramped up their exercise and mastered new eating patterns. They did get overuse injuries, but like pro athletes, they willingly "played through" aches and pains. Their weight came off fast and furious—actually, too fast in some cases—I had to temporarily pull some of the contestants off the program because, in an attempt to lose even more weight than I recommended, they were eating too little, avoiding carbs, exercising excessively, and lifting weights improperly. My approach was already aggressive enough, so when contestants went

11

overboard, it occasionally resulted in some blood test abnormalities. Luckily, no permanent damage occurred and they got better with rest and a few hundred more calories consumed.

Chapter Two

Fat-Loss Myths and New Scientific Discoveries

Scientific discoveries from reality TV? Is that an oxymoron? Can intelligence seep from unscripted television chatter? If you squeeze coal dust hard enough, will diamonds form?

Well, stuff happened! The television show, birthed by a clutch of brilliant show-biz types with nary a biology major between them, did indeed advance science. The show proved that if you motivate very overweight couch potatoes of both sexes and multiple ethnicities, they can lose gobs and gobs of fat safely over a short time span. The first 64 contestants averaged a staggering 60-plus-pound fat loss over five months—three times more than anticipated from the most rigorous medical diet plans (which average 20 pounds after one year)—while 21 alternates who didn't get cast on the show and were sent home without a road map didn't drop a single pound on average.

Far-greater-than-expected fat loss might not be a 10 on the Nobel Richter scale , but data from the initial *Biggest Loser* seasons did advance science by discrediting many weight-loss notions promulgated by stodgy, ivory-tower obesity researchers.

BELIEFS VERSUS FACTS

Belief # 1: Unfit overweight people are incapable of prolonged vigorous exercise.

New Scientific Fact: Shockingly, overweight, even morbidly obese couch potatoes are capable of exercising as long and as intensely as professional athletes!

True, at first they're slow as molasses, can't lift much weight, or slam dunk a basketball, but the 64 initial *Biggest Loser* contestants—ordinary working folks from every walk of life—did something previously thought impossible. They grunted through up to four hours of exercise a day, six days a week! And they came back for more. Sure, they were sore, mostly achy knees, calves, and feet, but they kept exercising. On a relative basis, they worked out every bit as hard as NFL players submitting to grueling two-a-day preseason practices.

Some exercise was vigorous, even on the edge of exhaustion. One contestant swore before the show that he worked out hard six hours a week, but I knew that was unlikely when his initial treadmill test showed no conditioning response. After the show, he leveled with me, saying he had spent a few nights dancing at clubs, but he now saw that the dancing was nothing compared to the intensity of his current workouts. Several morbidly obese male and female contestants—with well over 100 extra pounds of fat each—sometimes worked out six hours a day despite my pleas that this was overkill.

This capability is huge! It's massive! It opens a double door of opportunity, a brand-new option for fat reduction that simultaneously prevents or treats reams of obesity-related illnesses. It also directly contradicts the United States Surgeon General's recommendation for what I call "dumbed-down activity" for overweight Americans looking to attain a healthy weight: "Start with a 10-minute walk three times a week and work your way up to 30 minutes of brisk walking or other form of moderate activity five times a week." Unfortunately, this level of physical activity does not result in weight loss. Adherence to this exercise recommendation can't even prevent fat gain—or put a dent in their hypertension, hypercholesterol, or diabetic tendencies.

Belief # 2: Busy two-career overweight couples with kids have no time to exercise.

New Scientific Fact: When overweight families were committed to regular, at-home exercise, they universally adjusted to the extra two-plus hours of exercise by watching two-plus hours less of TV!

Talk about a paradox! A television show resulting in less TV viewing! But that's exactly what happened. The first 64 contestants watched zero television at the initial exercise boot camp, and when they settled into their weight-loss exercise routines when they got home—averaging a tad over two hours a day, six days a week—their TV viewing time dropped by almost two hours—from their preshow viewing habits of 2.75 hours a day to only one hour a day! An interesting comparison: The obese individuals selected as alternates for the first several seasons of the show (they never made it on the actual show) made no major changes in their TV viewing habits and didn't increase exercise or lose weight. (The relationship between the amount of TV viewing and obesity is nearly as strong as that between smoking and lung cancer!)

Other interesting changes occurred within the ranks of the initial 64 on-the-air contestants. These exercise converts learned to prioritize better. One 40-year-old neat freak working mom told me she'd learned to keep the kids' bedroom doors closed and drive the family car with a little dirt on the hood because after an hour of exercise before work and an hour after work, there was no longer time for picking up after her kids or weekend car washes. (There is, of course, another possible explanation: Exercise is a powerful treatment for those with obsessive-compulsive/clean-freak traits!)

Belief # 3: Introducing exercise to a weight-loss diet adds little to the eventual weight loss. The standard nutritionist's lecture line is that while an aggressive six-month diet can drop 5 to 10 percent of your weight, exercise adds little or, at most, a few extra percentage points.

15

New Scientific Facts:

- Two-a-day exercise together with moderate caloric restriction in motivated dieters yields three- to tenfold more fat loss than other documented diets.
- Exercising two times a day triggers fat-for-muscle exchanges and fluid shifts that complicate the interpretation of "scale weights."

If you lose 15 pounds on a diet, you naturally assume you lost all fat, and you naturally assume you're now healthier. Sorry, not true. You really haven't the foggiest idea how much of that 15 pounds was water, muscle, bone, or fat. Suffice it to say that with a standard fad or low-carb diet, lean tissue loss may be comparable to fat loss!

Low amounts of exercise don't increase the absolute number of pounds lost, but it may bump up the proportion of weight loss that is fat. Higher levels of exercise—as advocated in The WOW! ℞—together with moderate caloric restriction, not only melt away fat more quickly than diets alone, they ensure that muscle is gained or at least maintained.

After the initial exercise boot camp in Los Angeles, the average contestant continued to lose large amounts of fat by exercising at home six days a week for 2 to 2.5 hours each day. The oft-quoted articles claiming that exercise did not induce weight loss used puny exercise amounts, often in the range of walking half an hour a day. There's nothing wrong with a brief walk. I encourage it. If everyone in the world took those extra steps, it might be sufficient to slow weight gain and encourage people to progress to do more exerting activity; then in a generation or so, there'd be no obesity. But make no mistake, for an obese adult, a daily half-hour walk is not sufficient for weight loss. Nor is it sufficient to maintain weight after dropping 30 pounds of fat.

Belief # 4: Gastric bypass surgery is appropriate for morbidly obese adults and children (those with a body mass index [BMI] over 40) or just plain fat folks (BMI over 35) with worrisome diseases like diabetes, high blood pressure, arthritic hips or knees, or heart disease.

New Scientific Fact: Motivated massively obese and just plain obese individuals now have a new choice, a nonsurgical option they can do at home. The six-month and preliminary 18-month fat-loss numbers of The WOW! ℞ are equivalent to the results that patients get after gastric bypass! Approximately 175,000 gastric bypass surgeries are performed each year in the United States. It's life-prolonging intervention in expert hands, although after paying $25,000, there's still a 40 percent chance of major postoperative complications. In a less-experienced surgeon's hands, there's a whopping 3 percent chance of instant skin and bones—otherwise known as death! An alarming 11 percent of Medicare patients die after gastric bypass surgery! The reality is, gastric bypass is major, risky surgery requiring the utmost surgical skills for a group of patients who almost always have medical conditions that interfere with routine healing.

One of *The Biggest Loser* show's "beyond-morbidly-obese" contestants—who'd been urged by a reputable surgeon to have gastric bypass—was initially hesitant to sign on for the program. I helped convince him that even in his condition the exercise program was do-able. The most gratifying aspect of my association with *The Biggest Loser* was watching this individual shrink from an artery-clogging, lymph-blocking, vein-popping 51-percent body fat to an absolutely normal 22 percent. Sensational! And that wasn't all. I also got to see his energy level return to normal and the disappearance of his hypertension, sleep apnea, and crippling weight-related ankle and foot problems—for which another highly respected surgeon had recommended a complete joint fusion.

Belief # 5: High blood pressure warrants treatment with blood pressure meds, elevated glucoses require diabetic medication, gastroesophageal reflux merits treatment with acid-suppressing drugs, asthma should be treated with asthma inhalers, low energy and depression should be treated with antidepressants, and so forth.

17

New Scientific Fact: In overweight individuals, aggressive exercise and moderate caloric restriction is the first and best do-no-harm prescription for high blood pressure, adult onset diabetes, high cholesterol, depression, low energy, reflux, snoring, asthma, joint pains, or just plain feeling blah.

Improvements in the contestants' health were nothing short of miraculous. At the show's beginning, 48 percent of contestants had systolic hypertension (the top number of your blood pressure) and 58 percent had elevations in the diastolic (bottom number) that, if left untreated, would pose a significant risk for stroke or heart disease. They all met the criteria for taking medications to regulate their blood pressure. (As an aside, many had no idea they had high blood pressure and only a few were on treatment.) Fast forward to the show's completion: A mere 11 percent needed blood pressure medication! Even more gratifying, of the 19 percent who smoked at the onset of the program, over half remained off cigarettes at the two-year mark. . . and still managed to lose just as much fat as their peers!

Similarly, 25 percent started with prediabetic fasting sugar or insulin levels, but the diabetic-leaning levels resolved in all but 5 percent after their weight loss. There were also gratifying resolutions of gastro-esophageal reflux (33 percent affected before, only 3 percent afterward), snoring (47 percent with greatly annoyed partners before, down to only 18 percent after), and asthma (27 percent affected before, only 9 percent afterward). All contestants reported dramatic energy and mood enhancements; overall quality-of-life improvements; and more modest, but nonetheless significant, sparks on the sexual front—not to mention gratifying changes in sexual organ sizes of men; but more on that later.

Belief # 6: The recommended rate for losing weight safely is 1 to 2 pounds per week.

New Scientific Fact: Over the first several months, the recommended rate for losing fat safely is 1 to 2 percent of body weight per week.

A 2006 *Time* magazine health survey opined that safe levels of weight loss are 1 to 2 pounds a week. I've also seen this same false "wisdom" in several newspaper articles (some critical of *The Biggest Loser*). First off, how crazy is it to lump 5'-tall fat preteens in with 6' 4," 400-pound adult men? When discussing a safe rate for losing weight, you must talk in terms of percent of an individual's body weight, and you don't need to be a rocket scientist to know that you must separate water, bone, and muscle loss (all bad) from fat loss (the goal).

A 450-pounder can lose 4 to 5 pounds of fat a week merely by cutting back calories from 3,500 to 3,000 and adding an hour of intense exercise. And when it comes to "fake" weight loss, the sky's the limit: If he works out hard for 90 minutes in a hot environment (i.e., loses water and water heavy glycogen), he could easily drop 15 pounds (about 14.5 pounds of it water). Is that unsafe? No, not if he promptly rehydrates and adds back carbs.

In truth, many contestants registered huge weight loss numbers on the scale some weeks, little during others, often as a direct result of fluid shifts. Contestants on each of the first three *Biggest Loser* shows consistently lost over 4 to 8 pounds of fat per week over the initial several months, then settled in to lose on average just over 2.5 to 5 pounds of fat per week (a little over 1 percent of body weight) over the entire five- to eight-month weight-loss period. Was that unsafe? When done under a doctor's supervision, no. To be on the super-safe side, however, it makes sense to err on the side of caution when recommending a home plan for the general public.

Belief # 7: When you lose weight, expect 25 to 40 percent of the lost mass to be lean tissue; expect only 60 to 75 percent of the lost mass to be fat.

New Scientific Fact: *The Biggest Loser* experience proved—for the first time—that you can lose large amounts of weight in a relatively short period of time and essentially all of the weight lost can be fat!

An optimal fat-loss plan can get you as close to your WOW! weight in as short a time span as is safely possible while preserving and even building more muscle. This is, in fact, what The WOW! ℞ delivers. And by preserving or even augmenting calorie-guzzling, metabolism-escalating muscle—something one-note diets can't address—The WOW! ℞ puts you up front in the pole position for keeping the fat off.

Belief # 8: All weight loss is good; the method of weight loss is irrelevant.

New Scientific Fact: Weight loss is a double-edged sword.

True, the loss of stored (excess) fat has universal health benefits. However, the loss of essential fat (dropping below 3 to 5 percent body fat in men, or 12 to 15 percent in women), or the loss of muscle, bone, or fluid (remember that about 80 percent of a piece of muscle and 20 percent of a glob of fat tissue is salty water) is detrimental to our health. As a doctor, I've been taught to search for the visual cues of this type of detrimental weight loss as an early sign of cancer, chronic infections like HIV, or even depression. Hollowed eye sockets, sucked-in cheeks, sticky oral mucous, dry underarms, and atrophied arm, leg and facial muscles are flashing warning signs of disease. It's no wonder that "starvation" fad diets and aggressive low-carb or low-fat weight-loss diets without proper exercise make the dieter appear "sick." Why? Because they are sick! They've lost essential water, muscle, and bone!

Belief # 9: Overweight dieters should follow their progress by compulsively weighing themselves every day.

New Scientific Fact: Daily scale weights are misleading.

Scale weights are not particularly accurate. Comparison of two expertly calibrated doctor scales were found to occasionally vary by as many as 2 pounds; home scales, not infrequently, were off by 5 pounds, and in some instances, even 10.

Your weight may vary (up or down) by 5 to 15 pounds, depending on the time of day (or for women, the particular day of your period) the weight is taken, or your level of hydration, ankle swelling, and salt intake, or the amount of your liver and muscle glycogen supplies (vigorous exercise and carb depletion can acutely lower glycogen stores).

Scale weights do not reflect whether lower weight results from excess fat loss or from water, muscle, critical organ proteins, or bone loss. With regard to the typical low-carb diet: Initial lean tissue and water weight loss often delude dieters into thinking their goals are being met, but when eventual (necessary) water and glycogen replenishment results in weight gain of as many as 5 to 10 pounds, it's often depressing, sending dieters back into the arms of junk food.

Body weight can vary (up) when acclimating to vigorous exercise—a phenomena called hyperhydration. Four weeks into the initial *Biggest Loser* show, accurate body-fat analysis showed that the men and women alike had gained fluid weight! And their kidneys were still sending strong signals indicating the body was fluid depleted! What happened? First, the body makes a clever adjustment the instant someone begins vigorous exercise: It holds onto extra fluid inside the blood vessels to maximize heart contraction and the body's ability to thermoregulate (get rid of excess heat). The previously sedentary *Biggest Loser* contestants—who started strenuous workouts in the middle of a stifling California summer—exhibited this phenomenon in spades. However, several things happened that have never before been reported in the annals of weight-loss medicine. Number one, the extra fluid amounts were huge, over 10, and sometimes approaching 15 pounds, perhaps due to the large size of the contestants. Secondly, they gained this fluid in the blood while remaining "relatively" dehydrated! Obviously, these countercurrents make the interpretation of scale weights tough, if not impossible.

On episodes of *The Biggest Loser*, the contestants' scale-weight measurements were used for entertainment purposes, but their ongoing weight results in no way indicated what was really going on inside their bodies and with their health. For health monitoring, body-fat percentages and then eventually water, bone, and muscle levels were religously recorded. Unfortunately, confirming the accuracy of these state-of-the-art technologies, then fairly adjusting for age, gender, and ethnicity and next explaining it all to the TV audience would be a daunting task. The behind-the-scenes bickering about the best "health measurement" was itself high drama—almost worthy of its own show. Bottom line—I found once-a-week weights were as "motivating" as daily weights. And contestants learned to gauge their fat loss in belt-notch increments and to take their fluctuating weights with a grain of salt.

Belief # 10: Ninety-nine percent of people who lose large amounts of weight will gain it all (or more) back.

Early Indications Are This Could Eventually Be a New Scientific Fact: Individuals who lose fat and maintain muscle by regular exercise (together with moderate caloric restriction) can maintain weight loss forever.

Let's be honest, losing weight is really tough; maintaining it can be even tougher. But 99 percent recidivism (or weight regain)—which a hospital's head gastric bypass surgeon quoted to me—is not accurate for people who continue to exercise and stay conscious about healthy food choices.

A review of the world's medical literature reveals that successfully keeping weight off is literally impossible with diet alone. Worse yet, four to five years after the completion of every studied diet, not only was the weight gained back, but a third to two-thirds of the dieters gained even more weight compared to their starting point. The number-one predictor of success at weight maintenance is exercise and an active, physical lifestyle! So it came as no real surprise that *The Biggest Loser* contestants—with exercise becoming an integral part of their lives—maintained 80 percent of their weight loss, and fully half did not regain any weight two years after the start of the diet (10 of the first 64 members were unable to be reached).

Belief # 11: There is no magic pill for rapid weight loss. There is no magic pill for weight maintenance after significant weight loss.

New Scientific Fact: There is a magic pill for rapid fat loss: Two hours of daily exercise (plus moderate caloric restriction).

There is also a magic pill for weight maintenance after significant weight loss: one hour or more of vigorous daily exercise.

ONE MORE HURDLE

One vexing scientific hurdle remained: I could not logically conclude that the dramatic fat loss seen in virtually every *Biggest Loser* contestant was fully applicable to the average obese American. During the initial two months of the five- to eight-month shows (the original 10- to 12-week plan was drastically elongated once the network saw firsthand the drama involved in weight loss!), *Biggest Loser* contestants had a lot of help with their weight loss. Every bite of food was monitored 24/7 by TV cameras. They had exercise equipment available around the clock. They had fitness trainers organizing daily sessions and providing motivation. They had big-time money dangling in front of their noses—a chance for a quarter-of-a-million-dollar prize, to be exact. The financial incentives and handholding were substantially less for the 48 contestants on the spring 2006 *Biggest Loser Special Edition* shows (the family-versus-family shows).

Both their potential prize money and their filmed, personalized boot-camp instruction were far less than what *Biggest Loser-1* and *Biggest Loser-2* contestants received. But to my surprise, at the five-month mark, when the *Biggest Loser Special Edition* finale was filmed, despite lower prize money and less trainer face time, the contestants lost nearly as much weight as their *Biggest Loser-1* and *Biggest Loser-2* brethren!

Still, American medical journal editors were dubious, refusing to publish studies documenting the contestants' dramatic fat loss, averaging 35 percent of their original weights over eight months. They claimed this "fantasy weight-loss environment"—financial inducements with round-the-clock exercise with motivating trainers—was prohibitively expensive and, therefore, not applicable in the real world of weight loss; they also claimed the financial incentives made the research "unscientific" (despite the fact that many medical studies offer subjects payments of thousands of dollars just to participate). Although I disagreed, I had no proof that they were wrong either.

I racked my brain. I fought off Ghirardelli dark chocolate cravings. Where in the world could I get the millions of dollars needed to study a nationwide sampling of obese Americans who were following the road map of this dramatic fat-loss program, but with no TV cameras, no boot camp, no handholding trainers, and no financial incentives and compare them to our *Biggest Loser* TV contestants—not to mention a control group of people who would have no instructions of any kind?

The answer came the very next day.

Chapter Three

The WOW! ℞ Home Fat-Loss Team

"*Biggest Loser* casting wants us to block out three days," my secretary groaned over the intercom. "In two weeks, they've got 70 contestants flying in." At first I was slightly teed off—not that I'm ever particularly sunny at 6 P.M. with stacks of work and hospital rounds remaining. "You're all booked up. What should we do?"

I slumped back. Show-biz medicine was a fun diversion, but with its ever-changing and always-urgent needs, it was overwhelming at times, and booked or not booked, there was no way I could do 70 medical exams in three days. Obesity physicals are scary fishing expeditions, and these contestants were beyond obese—in many cases, beyond morbidly obese. The first 85 contestants who came through my doors for previous seasons had presented a veritable pathologic potpourri. Their hometown medical "clearances" notwithstanding, diseases I "allowed"— high blood pressure, diabetes, hypercholesterolemia, cigarette smoking, gastroesophageal reflux, and sleep apnea—were often in desperate need of treatment. Deal-breaker medical ailments—unstable heart disease, critical anemia, hypothyroidism, drug addiction, and pregnancy— occurred about five percent of the time. But it took exhaustive medical, psychological, orthopedic, and dietary exams, along with exotic labs, stress testing, and body fat and body fluid checks to ferret out each hidden medical land mine. Cut even one diagnostic corner? No way. Guaranteed, something would eventually explode.

Suddenly, I straightened up in my chair. Something my secretary said snapped me out of my worst-case worries. Something big was happening! For the usual show, casting would send me 20 hopefuls from which they'd select the final 14-member cast. Now, with the onset of the third year, there were 70 hopefuls. . . from a show that was always over budget?

"Get casting on the line."

That's when manna started falling from the sky.

GOING NATIONAL

In show business you have to keep reinventing yourself or things grow stale. The new slant for *The Biggest Loser-3* season, I found out, was to go nationwide. There would be one contestant from each of the 50 states. The show planned to fly out 70 hopefuls to fill those slots, and I knew from experience that every season those hopefuls were bigger and, therefore, sicker. Fourteen lucky individuals would be chosen to be on the regular NBC show, but here is where I went speechless—fortune this good rarely rained down, and this was a torrent! The 36 state representatives that didn't get chosen would still be encouraged to lose weight, but they wouldn't be kept on the ranch; they'd be sent home with no home gym equipment, no personal trainers, no diet services—just the lure that after four to ten weeks, one contestant would rejoin the televised show (basically a 1-in-36 chance of being one of 15 contestants in contention for the $250,000 prize). The show producers and I came up with a plan to keep them at their hotel in Los Angeles for an extra three days after they failed to make the show so I could conduct a crash course on exercise and diet.

It was almost ideal from my scientific research-oriented perspective. Fourteen test subjects got the blue-plate special; 36 got a three-day WOW! ℞ crash course and 20 alternates, not part of the 50 chosen state representatives, were sent home with no weight-loss road map whatsoever. I'd finally be able to scientifically document exactly what impact living in the ranch boot-camp environment would have; I'd be able to see if the 24/7 TV cameras really did make the boot camp folks more accountable, and just how much help were daily trainers and how much of a factor was that quarter-of-a-million-dollar carrot hung out in front of them. I'd finally be able to present weight-loss results scientists wouldn't be able to quibble with. Sure, even the 36 home participants were "extra" motivated by their association—however peripheral—with a TV show. But, their level of motivation could be reproduced quite simply in the "real world." If journal editors rejected this article, it would be for non-scientific reasons.

If the home contestants were capable of radical fat loss without hand-holding, it would have sweeping implications for tens of millions of obese Americans. There'd never before been a medical TV show with this amount of drama! What would the numbers say when these two groups squared off in two months time? Science is the ultimate reality show.

The Home Team Plan Takes Shape

Even the best-laid plans have glitches. The next night I actually inherited my 36 "subjects," they were beyond despondent; I had to remind myself that after a two- or three-month audition process, they'd just been passed over for a dream role as a TV show contestant. Frankly, I panicked. Had all the motivated, gung-ho types been selected for the show? Would the jilted 36 be in any mood to cooperate? Was this comparison fatally flawed?

But, for better or worse, there was no turning back. Over the preceding weeks, I had cobbled together a three-day crash course to force-feed the 36 leftover contestants the exercise and dietary basics every obese person who is serious about losing weight must master—the basic WOW! ℞. I had assembled a fat-fighter team: a registered dietician, a weight-loss psychologist, and an athletic trainer, while I filled the shoes of the motivating running coach and weight-loss doctor. We'd follow up with the 36 by rotating participation in weekly phone calls and mini-newsletters. Although the fat-fighter team looked great on paper, it was not to be. The former professional football athletic trainer I'd recruited to help spot and treat injuries early on was needed full-time for the TV contestants and not available to the 36 home contestants. The show had no budget for the extra costs my weight-loss program would incur, so they inked a sponsorship deal with a fitness chain, and in return, the fitness chain understandably expected they would handle the exercise side of the crash course. I panicked again when I received their workout plans for my morbidly obese couch potatoes.

Talk about an education! Like every fitness chain in the country, their workout philosophies were worlds apart from mine. I believe there's overwhelming evidence showing that our circadian (24-hour) clock can be a huge help if we stick to regular exercise and eating patterns. Obviously, a key objective was to drill home to my undisciplined overweight charges the essential nature of habitual 5:30 A.M. and 5:00 P.M. workouts (or whatever regular times best fit with the exercisers' schedules). But fitness chain trainers are busy with their personal clients during those optimal peak hours, and, in this instance, proposed splitting my 36 into groups of 12 and rotating through the limited number of aerobic machines and weight-lifting stations at different times each day for each group.

I wanted to use nature to motivate the 36, to run four miles every sunrise from their Manhattan Beach hotel to the *Baywatch* beach and lifeguard stations. But fitness chains like to use aerobic sessions to familiarize clients with state-of-the-art treadmills and elliptical machines often depressingly crammed side by side, complete with fields of flashing red lights indicating misleading "fat-burning" heart rate zones.

My goals were to establish a routine, maximize the number of calories burned per hour, given the time constraints faced by the busy average American, and do it as cheaply as possible. The fitness chain wanted improved endurance and strength, but they had no plan for optimizing fat loss in woefully out-of-shape subjects. They wanted to introduce novice exercisers to machines and trainers. I felt that more cost-effective, invigorating, natural, and serene options exist.

Exhibits 3.1 and 3.2 compare the differences, as I see them, between typical fitness-chain workout philosophies and mine:

Exhibit 3.1 Fitness-Chain Workout Philosophy

- Workout time: When trainer has time; when class is available.
- Location: Gymbased, indoors.
- Travel time: Yes (can be mitigated by biking or running to gym as your warm-up).
- Cost: Expensive.
- Environmental cost: Yes (gas for travel to gym, electricity for machines).
- Aerobics: Machines (treadmills, elliptical, stair-stepper, stationary bike, etc.).
- Strength Exercises: Gym-based machines.
- Goals: Improving endurance and strength, encouraging use of exercise machines only big gyms can afford.

Benefits:
- Motivation from "group" environment.
- Motivation and injury-prevention advice from well-qualified personal trainers.
- Possible dating opportunities for singles.
- Stationary bike may be only suitable initial pre-weight loss exercise for morbidly obese exerciser (legs don't rub).

Downside:
- Some trainers are not adequately qualified and give clients misleading exercise information.

Downsides of Gym Machine Aerobics:
- Noise pollution.
- Treadmill is inferior exercise compared with outdoor running.
- As a rule, individuals self-select lower-intensity exercise levels on exercise machines as compared to walk-running.
- Inaccurate calorie-burning information on machines.
- Infectious disease concerns.

Downsides of Gym Machine Strength Training:
- Machine strength training does not maximize calorie burn (too few muscles working simultaneously).
- Machine strength training does little to develop balance.
- One body part machine strength training poorly simulates real life situations where total body muscle synergy is needed.
- Machine strength training equipment is "overwhelming" to novices.
- Infectious disease concerns.

Exhibit 3.2 The WOW! ℞ Workout Philosophy

- Workout time: At exactly the same time each day (the time most convenient for the exerciser).
- Location: Homebased, primarily outdoors.
- Travel time: No.
- Cost: Inexpensive.
- Environmental cost: None.
- Aerobics:

  Nature (running, hiking, swimming, biking, stair climbing)
  Recreational sports
  Aerobic machines as fallback option
- Strength exercises: Home-based free weights and ankle/wrist weights.
- Goals: Fat loss, cost effectiveness, time effectiveness.

Benefits:

- Regular exercise time puts circadian rhythm in sync, helping to optimize sleep, exercise, and work abilities.
- Mood elevation (from high lux natural sunlight).
- Builds self-starter instincts (in all life aspects).
- Running or brisk walking provides optimal serene milieu for self-reflection.
- Absence of "workout" group atmosphere, which some individuals feel is implicitly "judgmental" about their bodies.

Downside:

- Aerobic machines are best to rehabilitate leg injuries. A stationary bike or elliptical is invaluable when one is recovering from foot, shin, calf, or knee injuries.

Secret Ingredients

Suffice it to say, I took over the running coach's role and we used the fitness chain's trainers for teaching body weight and Swiss Ball exercises. No question, my original intent was to secure a fitness trainer for each home contestant for several weeks to help implement my running and free-weight workout instructions, especially the resistance moves some of the women who'd never touched a dumbbell struggled with. But the TV show's budget was threadbare and didn't allow for trainers past the first few days' crash seminar. Since we knew that some contestants couldn't afford trainers, in fairness we told every contestant that personal trainers were strictly verboten, and participants would be summarily tossed off the show if we found out they'd used one. So an entirely new component of the experiment was born. Namely, how important is the personal trainer's role for ultimate success on this aggressive exercise-based fat-loss plan? Up to this point, every academic medical study subject adhering to high levels of exercise and all prior *Biggest Loser* boot-camp participants had access to the services of round-the-clock trainers. Now I'd be able to gauge the impact: Was it a key component or not? What exactly were the secret ingredients for dramatic fat loss?

THE HOME TEAM

I was giddy with anticipation. Would the underdog at-home contestants be able to keep up with the dramatic weight-loss numbers of the ranchers? And who exactly were these at-home contestants (see Table 3.1)?

Quick Observations About the 36 States Home Team

The following observations also hold true for all of the 172 *Biggest Loser* participants:

- The women had lower body mass indexes (BMI, which is weight (lbs) × 703 ÷ height (in)²), but much higher body-fat percentages than the men (i.e., proof that the BMI is a second-class indicator of true body composition).
- The women carried excess fat around their waists, but relatively

Table 3.1 *The Biggest Loser* Home Team Statistics

	Women (Averages)	Men (Averages)
Age	31	34
Height (inches)	65	71
Weight at age 21	188	247
Weight one year previously△	231	321
Weight at beginning of show	243	339
Body Mass Index (BMI)	40	47
WOW! weight (pounds)	158 (25% BF) (118 lean + 40 fat)	222 (15% BF) (189 lean + 33 fat)
Ideal weight loss (pounds)	85	117
Ideal weight loss (percent)*	34.6%	34.5%
Waist at belly button (inches)	51	53
Hips (inches)	52	56
Body Fat (percent)		
Bod Pod	51	45
iDEXA	50	44
Calipers	43	38
RMR ("ready-made" Mufflin equation)	1,810	2,490
RMR (from percent body-fat test)	1,560	2,256
Pre-show exercise per week (hours)	3.1	2.3

△Studies show that overweight individuals significantly underestimate their true weights.
*Weight loss needed to get to WOW! weight.

more on the back of their arms and hips compared to the men.
- On average, the self-reported two to three weekly hours of moderate (walking level) exercise in this group before embarking on The WOW! ℞ did not result in weight loss; it did not even prevent weight gain.

- *The Biggest Loser* finalists needed to lose, on average, 33 percent of their body weights to reach their ideal WOW! weights.
- The percentage of weight loss needed to achieve WOW! weight was equal for the men and the women. Although the women started off with higher body-fat percentages, the ideal body-fat percentage for a man is 10 percent lower than a woman's (ideal body fat is about 15 percent for men, 25 percent for women).

All Contestant Hopefuls Were Overweight, and Most Were Also Unhealthy

Most of the finalists who made it through the screening process were unhealthy when they arrived at *The Biggest Loser* production offices in Los Angeles. But guess what? Neither the TV producers nor the potential contestants had any idea! Sure, everyone knows obese and deconditioned individuals harbor hidden disease, but the extent of the contestants' heartburn, asthma, depression, and sleep apnea, as well as whacked-out blood pressure, blood sugar, insulin, cholesterol, and inflammatory markers, was alarming, and it never registered with the contestants (or even some of their doctors).

On their entrance questionnaires, just 13 percent of *The Biggest Loser-3* applicants reported a history of high blood pressure. However, when they were examined in my office, 71 percent sent the mercury monometer to abnormal heights! Likewise, only 3 percent acknowledged diabetic or pre-diabetic conditions, yet the lab exams revealed fully 31 percent were either undiagnosed full-on diabetics (7 percent) or prediabetics (24 percent)! Most had no idea what an inflammatory marker was (it's a hormone that fat produces that reflects inflammation, which, in turn, is closely linked to blood vessel damage), but a third of the applicants had spikes that would convince Vegas oddsmakers to bet on an early stroke or heart attack.

Despite all that, I'm proud to say that every medically cleared contestant was very successful. Sure, we had our share of wear-and-tear orthopedic injuries, but 98 percent of the participants finished the program strong, losing significant amounts of fat, getting truly fit, gaining new energy, expanding life horizons, and adding an average of five to nine years to their life spans. Not a bad deal for six to eight months of feel-good exercise that didn't interfere with work or cost more than two hours a day of TV viewing time.

How the Home Team Compared to Those on the Ranch

The initial fat-loss numbers for The WOW! ℞ Home Team were looking promising, but it was just too early to tell. Then lo and behold, at the two-month mark, a jaw-dropping trend emerged! Despite no significant prize money, no live-in weight-loss ranch, no personalized training, no home exercise equipment, no time away from family or work, no 24/7 TV cameras to force accountability, the home contestants were losing 85 percent as much weight as the ranch contestants! Even more amazing was the fact that most home contestants appeared to be working out only half as many hours a day as their boot-camp brethren! I repeat: The home folks, including the top four female and top four male representatives who easily bested their ranch peers, were in some cases working out only half as many hours a day as the on-air boot-camp contestants!

I was flabbergasted. Everyone affiliated with the show was in shock. Had we stumbled on the "fat-burn" sweet spot, the mythical point where tolerable exercise (working out intensely 2 to 2.5 hours a day) and diet (just enough carb "kindling" to keep the fat "logs" blazing, just enough protein to keep the muscle from breaking down) intersect to maximally melt storage fat? Was there a secret home ingredient? A happier, more active home life outside of the daily intense workouts? Were boot-camp contestants dehydrating before high-pressure national TV weigh-ins and stunting fat loss? Or were they being overtrained, with counterproductive metabolic consequences?

I'll return to these fascinating medical mysteries later. For now, the real questions are simply: Can anyone follow the home teams' path to success? Can any motivated obese or even morbidly obese person get back into their thin clothes. . . and their lives? More to the point, can you do it?

Yes, you can! It's not jaw wiring. . . or stomach stapling! The top eight at-home 36 state representatives were able to lose more weight than the top eight live-in ranch contestants, but didn't have to exercise for nearly as long. . . and neither do you!

Let's get started!

Chapter Four

Getting Started!

WHY YOU MUST GET FIT AND LOSE FAT

Before I tell you about the actual WOW! ℞, you've got to get educated about obesity risks and then get motivated to lose fat. There are two basic approaches to losing fat:

1. The emotional gut-instinct approach: Stand in front of a plain wall and have a family member, friend, or your doctor take front, side, and back bathing suit photos of you from exactly six feet away. Put these pictures up on your bathroom mirror and refrigerator. Is this you?
2. The intellectual approach: Statistically speaking, 40-year-old "healthy" (i.e., no heart disease or diabetes yet) obese individuals die an average seven years prematurely—almost 20 percent of their remaining life! Young obese individuals are on track to have between 10 to 20 years of life prematurely lopped off. And the bad news doesn't stop there. These gruesome statistics are based on comparisons with "normal" weight folks—those with BMIs from 19 to 25—but doctors have now discovered that as many as half these folks have iceberg obesity, they're thin on the outside but fat on the inside, they possess metabolically dangerous levels of fat marbled around and into their livers and other abdominal organs. So the comparison group is flawed—and the risks of obesity may be even greater!

Is exercise two hours per day for six months impractical?
Would you encourage a loved one to attend two hours or more of outpatient rehab per day if you discovered they had a heroin habit? Would you expect your mom to agree to four hours of dialysis every other day if her kidneys failed? Would you take chemo two hours per day for six months if it could cure your newly diagnosed cancer?

If you have overflowing abdominal fat, you're facing a choice, in my opinion, not terribly dissimilar from the above examples. Your excess fat is a deliberate poison. It's not easy, but two hours per day of exercise with calorie counting and moderate caloric restriction for six months is a small price to pay to remove the poison.

You must choose between health and illness, energy and lethargy, life and death.

Find Your Motivation

Write down every reason you have to get fit and lose fat. This is my order of importance. What's yours?

- Feel better
- Live disability free
- Live longer
- Prevent disease
- Treat disease
- Improve mood
- Look better
- Be more athletic

(Okay, maybe when I was younger these last two were really at the top of the list.)

The "Not If But When" List

Think about how the following medical complications of excess fat are affecting your life (and the lives of your loved ones):

- Type-2 (adult-onset) diabetes mellitus and its complications (renal, ophthalmologic, neurological, and vascular)
- Hypertension
- High levels of bad cholesterol
- Low levels of good cholesterol
- Atherosclerotic cardiovascular disease
- Heart failure
- Hyperthermia
- Sticky platelets
- Arterial and venous blood clots
- Fatty liver disease, sometimes progressing to cirrhosis
- Gallstones
- Pancreatitis
- Infertility
- Birth defects (in infants born to obese mothers)
- Sleep apnea
- Asthma
- Nutritional deficiencies
- Gastroesophageal reflux disease
- Varicose veins
- Edema
- Alzheimer's disease
- Strokes
- Headaches
- Physical imbalance
- Vertebral disk disease
- Depression
- Anxiety and panic

- Binge eating
- Reactive bulimia
- Arthritis of weight-bearing joints (spine, hip, knee, ankle, and foot)
- Endometrial cancer
- Breast cancer
- Ovarian cancer
- Cervical cancer
- Prostate cancer
- Colorectal cancer
- Esophageal and throat cancer
- Gallbladder cancer
- Pancreatic cancer
- Renal cell cancer
- Stretch marks
- Boils, skin and nail infections
- Bags under the eyes
- Abnormal odors
- Skin ulcers
- Inaccurate diagnostic tests—CAT and MRI scans, bone density tests, stress thallium treadmill tests—or worse yet, the physical inability to even fit into the scanner
- Increased surgical risks
- Lower surgical success rates

Major Obstacles to Successful Fat Loss

Some major obstacles to fat loss include:

Lack of a Legitimate Road Map
There are many, many ways to lose weight, but precious few ways to

lose fat, not muscle, bone, and water and establish a lifelong routine that will significantly increase the chance of keeping the fat off long term.

Ignorance

It's worth repeating: People try to lose weight to get healthy, but they've got it inside out and backward. You need to lose fat, not "weight," and you've got to get healthy (first) to lose fat.

Depression

Among *The Biggest Loser* contestants, depression was overwhelmingly the number one cause of difficulty while trying to lose their excess fat. Depression affects perhaps 15 percent of the general adult population, but it runs closer to 40 percent or more in obese individuals.

Other psychological issues that can derail weight loss include anxiety, obsessive-compulsive tendencies, and binge-eating disorders. In addition, other obstacles include medical and orthopedic diseases, alcoholism, genetics, environment, and sleep deprivation.

What's Out There Now to Lose Weight?

Boil down the hundreds of diets floating in cyberspace and find only 10 choices—interestingly, none until now places a significant emphasis on vigorous exercise:

1. Diets that allow you to eat as much as you want (but limit certain foods): low-carbohydrate, low-glycemic index, low-fat diets; no processed foods, no white foods, no fruit, all fruit, all raw foods, etc.
2. Limit-what-you-eat diets (count calories, count points, portion control, willpower, liquid meal replacements, eat only pre-packaged or catered diet foods)
   - Moderate caloric restriction (within 10 to 20 percent of your estimated resting metabolic rate—the number of calories

you'd burn if you stayed in bed all day)
- Severe caloric restriction (less than 1,000 calories per day)
- Starvation (less than 500 calories per day)

3. Surgeon General "weight-loss" exercise: brisk walking for 30 minutes a day, three to six times per week
4. Weight-loss pills
   - Proven medications
   - Off-label use of one of other medications not approved for use as weight-loss pills
   - Stuff advertised on late-night television or spread via junk e-mail
5. Bariatric surgery (such as gastric-bypass surgery)
6. Weight-loss exercise
7. Diet plus Surgeon General exercise
8. Diet plus Surgeon General exercise plus weight-loss pills
9. Diet plus Surgeon General exercise plus bariatric surgery
10. Weight-loss exercise and moderate caloric restriction: The WOW! ℞

The Downside to Weight-Loss Options

What is the downside to these different weight-loss options? Some negatives include:

Diets

Diets don't work, period! Short term, any of the above diets can work, but typical results are marginal at best. When the Atkins, Zone, Weight Watchers, and Ornish diets were studied at Tufts University by Dr. Michael Dansingor, the current nutritional consultant to *The Biggest Loser*, weight loss at one year averaged just 2 to 3 percent, or 5 percent when hooked up with more aggressive education efforts. The findings were nearly identical in a second 2007 *Journal of American Medical*

Association study. A 5- to 10-pound weight loss is enough to secure some health benefits, but not enough to see physical change.

More importantly, even when a diet does work, the bigger question is: Will you keep the weight off? After several years, weight loss by diet alone, without exercise, is most likely to result in eventual weight gain, not successful weight maintenance! Perhaps the most poignant example is Oprah Winfrey's experience with the very low-calorie diet, Optifast, in 1988. She successfully lost 67 pounds in four months by drinking only the low-calorie shakes and taking supplements, and proudly showed off her new body in the fall of 1988. Sadly, as soon as she went off the diet, she regained all the weight she'd lost (gaining 10 pounds in the first two weeks alone). She has since referred to this liquid fast as an "iconic mistake."

Exercise

Unfortunately, exercise at the Surgeon General's recommended levels results in little, if any, real weight loss. Remember, the contestants chosen for *The Biggest Loser* were already reporting two to three hours per week of exercise at baseline—clearly not enough to make a dent in their fat!

Bottom line, when it comes to controlling fat—and health in general—a little exercise is good, more is better.

Weight-loss Pills

As of today, no FDA-approved product has reliably made much of a difference. Xenical and its recently approved half-strength over-the-counter offspring Alli, block the absorption of about a fourth of the fat you eat without any effect on the digestion of carbohydrates (including sugar) or protein. It would be great if you could just take a fat blocker before meals three times a day and start losing fat. Unfortunately, despite all the fanfare when Xenical was released in 1999, I observed no such miracles, only red-faced patients who had ignored my warnings that a fat, rich meal might lead to hard-to-control gas or brown oily spotting—or worse.

Meridia

Meridia, a stimulant that acts on brain neurotransmitters, has modest appetite-suppression effects, but when studied with a low-calorie diet, only 60 to 70 percent of a 23-pound weight loss was fat! As you might imagine, there exists an array of anti-seizure, anti-psychiatric, and migraine prophylactic drugs that anecdotally decrease appetite. Some patients and their doctors experiment with these drugs, alone or in combinations, but the jury is still out. Unfortunately, even if another potent Phen-Fen-like weight-loss potion is uncovered, you would have to take it for the rest of your life or risk regaining the weight. Remember when Phen-Fen was recalled because of possible cardiac complications? Former pill users went into overdrive making up for missed meals; many of them actually ended up heavier! But if doctors elect to prescribe pills for a lifetime to prevent this ugly weight recidivism, especially pills brawny enough to fool the brain's most basic drive, you've got to be fearful about side effects.

Bariatric Surgery

Bariatric surgery, formerly a last-ditch option for the morbidly obese, is now being performed on hundreds of thousands of individuals who qualify based on an arbitrary BMI number that may bear only scant resemblance to actual body-fat levels. And these surgeries are being performed without first exploring aggressive exercise and diet options; the doctors of many *Biggest Loser* contestants recommended stomach-stapling surgery even though none exercised more than 2 to 3 hours per week while restricting calories. One contestant was actually admitted to the hospital and was literally being wheeled to surgery before changing her mind and signing out AMA (against medical advice) based on a subconscious premonition that she'd find a better way to get down to her ideal weight...which she did!

The fact that bariatric surgery can be lifesaving under some conditions is largely overshadowed by an unacceptable death rate (0.5 percent at the "best" centers, 3 percent at less expert centers with up to 11% in Medicare seniors!) and a plethora of serious post-op complications, from immediate post-op bowel leaks to later metabolic problems to a lifelong increased risk of tuberculosis, increasing the already substantial base price of $25,000 to as much as $50,000.

And now there's a new trend: gastric bypass for teens. An October 2006 *New England Journal of Medicine* article—usually a trusted beacon of information—rubber-stamped bypass surgery on a teen with no reported body-fat determination who was exercising only three hours a week! Gosh, my 15 year old—like all her teammates—routinely works out 10-plus hours a week on the soccer and track teams, and we know obese kids can put in the same effort with proper coaching. Please! Let's give our kids a chance with weight-loss exercise and moderate caloric restriction under the watchful eyes of motivating coaches and sports doctors, as well as their parents, before exposing them to a life of metabolic and surgical risks!

Perhaps most importantly, even gastric-bypass surgery cannot lead to permanent weight loss without a significant diet and exercise plan. People desperate for a solution to their obesity often see the dramatic weight loss that occurs in the first year and think that the surgery will be an easy fix for them. What they don't realize is that gastric-bypass surgery patients are only successful at keeping the weight off long term when they drastically change their lifelong eating and exercise habits— otherwise, they, too, are at risk to regain a sizable portion, or all, of the weight lost.

So, the question is: If you have to dramatically change your eating habits and incorporate daily exercise into your life after gastric-bypass surgery in order to be successful long term, why not just change your habits now and avoid the risk of surgery?

The WOW! ℞: Try This First

Two years after starting on The WOW! ℞, *The Biggest Loser* home and TV contestants are, weight-wise, where they'd be expected to be if they had undergone bariatric surgery. Although many more people need to be studied on The WOW! ℞ for longer lengths of time before absolute scientific comparisons to bariatric surgery can be made, you don't need to be a rocket scientist, a bariatric surgeon, or the person footing the surgery bills to know which one you should try first.

Chapter Five

The WOW! ℞—Step-by-Step Guide

If you want to be successful in school, sports, business, or life you've got to have a coherent plan and a strong will; you've got to have near- and long-range goals and be fired up to meet the challenges ahead. Winning at weight loss is no different.

Here are the five cornerstone goals of The WOW! ℞, followed by step-by-step guidelines:

The WOW! ℞—CORNERSTONE GOALS

1. Get Fit

Ten thousand years ago, survival required huge amounts of physical exertion to hunt and forage—maybe the equivalent of a 20-mile walk-jog each day. Though our hunter-gatherer ancestors are long gone, the Amish, eschewing most modern technology, give us an inkling as to our physical capabilities. The Amish toil for seven (women) to nine (men) hours a day plowing fields, baling hay, or washing clothes by hand. Incidentally, their obesity rate is about one tenth ours despite a relatively high-fat diet. It's time for you to get fit; sure, you may not look or feel much like an athlete right now, but believe me, you've inherited the requisite walk-jog abilities. The payoff today for physical activity is not food; it's being smarter, happier, leaner, functionally younger, and gaining years of disease-free life.

2. Get Lean (Lower Storage Fat)

Once fit—and healthy—turn your attention here. Lose 10 to 15 percent of your starting weight in the first eight to ten weeks and make sure you lose fat—not muscle, essential enzymes, bone, electrolytes, or water. The more storage fat you have, the higher your risk for disease and early death. Fat—especially when marbled inside the abdomen—is not an inert blob as we naively thought years ago, but an angry endocrine organ spewing out hormonal messages fostering cancer, arteriosclerosis, hypertension, inflammation, diabetes, blood clotting, and lipid abnormalities. Losing fat is not the only route to ideal "leanness;" muscle development is an alternate path to improved health. Muscle loss is typical as we age, unless we do something to prevent it. Some of us with "iceberg obesity," despite a normal clothed exterior appearance, have, as mentioned before, a surprising excess of fat; others, however, have an elevated-percent body fat based on a paucity of muscle and, often, bone. This is not good in more ways than one. Not only does muscle burn many more calories than fat, it's also essential for generating feel-good, IQ-elevating brain chemicals and protecting the skeletal structure from injury. The initial goal of a thin "atrophied" person with iceberg obesity is not weight loss, it's muscle and bone gain!

3. Eat Right

No one needs much convincing when it comes to buying clean fuel to protect his or her car engine. Many people take better care of their cars than they do their own bodies—overdosing on sugar, processed grains, saturated and trans fats, the equivalent of sand-laced gasoline. Other dangerous "grocery-store" additives include cigarettes and other tobacco products, excessive alcohol, as well as mercury, PCBs, nitrites and nitrates. The old adage "you are what you eat" is a little over the top, but your dietary choices are key. High vegetable, fruit, and lean protein diets can moderate the risk of high blood pressure, cancer, heart disease, and obesity. This stands in stark contrast to recent vitamin C, E, and beta-carotene supplementation studies, where no disease prevention was found, and, in fact, possible harm identified by the indiscriminant use of these compounds.

4. Sleep Right

Keep a regular bedtime and wake-up time. There's a very real connection between sleep patterns, energy levels, and weight. Late-night shift workers are more likely to gain weight. Middle-aged women who sleep five or fewer hours per night are a third more likely to gain harmful levels of weight than their peers who sleep seven or more hours. Try this: start going to bed and waking up (and exercising) at the same time everyday. Based on my observations of my overworked, fatigued patients, a regular schedule can pay almost instant health dividends.

5. Stay on the program!

Stay on the program until you hit your WOW! weight (approximately two to three months if you're overweight, around four to eight months if you're obese, six to 12 months if morbidly obese). Next, ease into the MAINTAIN! Plan with its once-a-day exercise (what will you do with all that free time now?) and weekly monitoring (page 270)—for the rest of your life.

GETTING STARTED

Step 1: The Pre-participation Medical Exam for Hidden Medical-Psychological Disease

The 172 *Biggest Loser* contestants I saw for initial medical evaluations at my office were all young and attractive, with strong personalities. But percolating just below the surface of their hale-and-hearty exteriors were medical volcanoes primed to explode: undetected hypertension, diabetes, gastroesophageal reflux disease, asthma, elevated lipids, edema, sleep apnea, or early heart disease. And those were the people I medically approved to take part in the TV show! Also, despite the fact that all of the contestants I examined were chosen by the show from thousands of other obese applicants primarily on the basis of their outgoing, vivacious personalities, many silently suffered from severe depression, anxiety, nocturnal binging, even alcoholism—and I had no idea until months later. Ironically, some had gained additional weight as a complication of psychological medications they'd been prescribed for depression, which stemmed from their being overweight!

Bottom line, for safety's sake, you must have a thorough medical examination (Physician Screening Physical Exam in Section Three) to determine whether your current physical condition is adequate to permit you to embark on this life-transforming program centered on exercise. Plus, you will need to be monitored by your physician, who will be your medical ally to call if problems arise.

Take the home depression screen (see Section Three). If you score positive—as have many *Biggest Loser* participants—get the name of a first-rate psychologist and set up a consultation. Do not be penny-wise and pound-foolish! Even if your mood is not at basement levels, a consultation would be well worth it if your mind repeatedly trips up your well-intentioned weight-loss efforts. I don't want to jump ahead too much, but while "only" 15 percent of the participants felt as though they were depressed at the beginning, after two months and at the end of the show, when all of the contestants realized how radically better they felt, 55 percent reanalyzed the past and admitted that they had been significantly depressed on day one!

Step 2: Assemble "Fat-Fighter" Coaches and Teammates

You've already selected your doctor, now you need to staff the remainder of your team.

- If you can afford it, I highly recommend that you start with a dietitian. You need at least two lessons in calorie counting and a review session on shopping and tricks for preparing food in advance.
- A weight-loss psychologist is needed if depression or other previously hidden quirks become obvious as comfort foods are withdrawn. (Be honest with yourself in your thought journal!)
- A personal trainer can make sure you're pushing yourself to personal limits during your AM walk-jog and that you're properly performing your PM Push-Pull-Twist training. Two to three initial instruction sessions are best; I also suggest you arrange to have one final refresher session at the two-month mark.
- Enlist a family member (or figure out how to use the self-timer on your camera) to get monthly front, side, and back pictures, as well as weekly video clips of you verbalizing the ups and downs of your fat-loss journey. It makes for one great home motivational movie; it may be of great use during the maintenance phase.
- Lastly, recruit solid teammates. Ask neighbors, coworkers, or family members (including your kids) if they want to join you and lose excess fat and enhance their looks, energy, and health. Friendly wagers may give an extra boost to some people. Work out together when able, talk out problems, brag about milestones via e-mails, and circulate new weights. Someone too embarrassed to give out their weight or photograph their belly—like an alcoholic who hides the bottles—is not yet ready for this program.

Step 3: Get "Before" Photographs and Videotapes of Yourself

Front, back, and side bathing suit pictures are a wake-up call; they chronicle the sum total of millions of bad choices and excuses—some personal, some societal. Besides—I've found, somewhat surprisingly, that pictures not only motivate, they also liberate. Once individuals acknowledged the photos, standing on a scale and facing up to the weekly weight became small potatoes.

Step 4: Determine Your Current Fat Weight

Obtain an accurate body composition analysis (fat tissue + lean tissue = body weight). This is an invaluable asset, providing a baseline against which you'll measure the impressive amounts of body fat that you'll be losing and also giving you accurate numerical facts about your body that will allow you to customize your WOW! ℞ to meet your individual needs.

Body weight alone is misleading. The bathroom scale can't tell the difference between gaining 5 pounds of fat or 5 pounds of muscle. The scale can't tell the difference between gaining 5 pounds of water during your period or gaining 5 pounds of fat. The scale can't stop you from bragging that you've kept your weight about the same over the last 10 years—when, in fact, you've gained 15 pounds of fat and lost 15 pounds of muscle!

The single best health index is an accurate body composition measurement differentiating fat from lean tissue. Newer technologies go further—dissecting how much of your lean tissue is bone (documenting bone health) and how much is water, both inside and outside of your cells (documenting your exact level of hydration). What is the silver lining of accurate body composition analysis? It's a phenomenal motivational tool. Many of my patients shriek when they read the number of pounds of body fat they're carrying around, and they're flabbergasted to see their body-fat images. An accurate body-fat analysis gives you several advantages: Since your resting metabolic needs (the number of calories you burn when you're sitting around inactively or at rest) are essentially all based on the amount of your lean (fat-free) tissue, when the body fat percentage of your weight is known, your individualized resting daily energy expenditure (RDEE) can be estimated; this, in turn, allows you to determine how many calories you should consume a day in order to achieve optimal fat loss.

Knowing the body-fat percentage of your weight also allows for an accurate prediction of your WOW! weight: Ideal body-fat for men is roughly 12 to 18 percent, for women it's around 22 to 27 percent. As a comparison, professional athletes are usually at 3 to 15 percent (men) and 15 to 22 percent (women), depending on their sport. Professional models and sex-symbol movie stars tend to range around 12 to 17 percent (men) and 19 to 27 percent (women), with models at the lower end, and actors and actresses at the higher end of these body-fat ranges.

In today's world, there are four methods for calculating body-fat percentage with adequate accuracy:

1. A DEXA (Dual Energy X-ray Absorptiometry) scan, which uses X-rays to distinguish fat from bone and all other fat-free tissue, is probably the most accurate generally available method. Unfortunately, it loses accuracy when a person's weight approaches 250 to 300 pounds, it's relatively expensive (several hundred dollars), and many physicians are not trained in interpreting these body-composition results. Although the DEXA is an X-ray machine, it emits only trivial radiation (equivalent of a coast-to-coast plane flight or 1/10 of a chest X-ray). However, even this small amount of radiation exposure means that women should not be tested if there is any chance of pregnancy.

   A newer (more expensive) iteration of DEXA, iDEXA (intelligent Dual Energy X-ray Absorptiometry), accommodates any body type up to 425 pounds and tells you visually the exact location of your excess fat (legs vs. arms vs. trunk vs. waist vs. buttocks). This

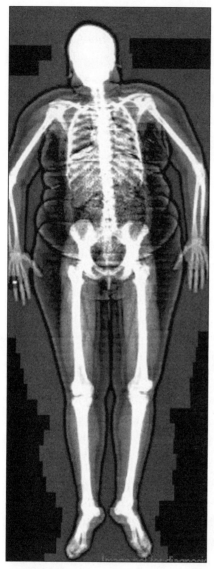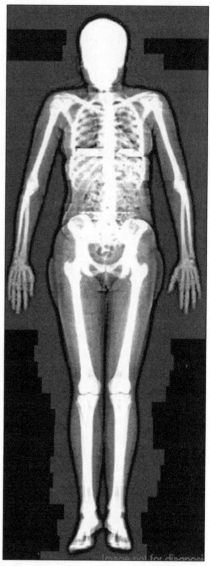

Could these pre- and post-WOW! ℞ iDEXA refrigerator door pinups influence your exercise and nutrition habits?

is critical info because excess belly fat (centripetal or android fat) has been linked to higher rates of heart disease than buttocks-hip fat. While iDEXA machines are not yet widely available, DEXA machines can be found in most cities.

2. Hydrostatic weighing involves an unpleasant 15-second underwater dunk after exhaling a full breath while sitting on a submerged scale. It's the time-honored method to determine body-fat percentage, but independent test sites are currently difficult to locate. Some physical education departments or university research centers offer it for around $50.

3. The Bod Pod (air displacement plethysmography) is a simple, reasonably priced (about $100) giant egg-shaped device used to determine the exact volume of the body. This is combined with a scale weight to get the body density (volume/weight). Since the density of fat, water, and muscle are known, equations exist to estimate body-fat percent. There are a few glitches; the lean-tissue density is affected by age, ethnicity, and hydration status; you cannot be Bod Pod tested after a workout or warm shower; and folks heavier than 400 pounds can't be squeezed into the egg. Given those caveats, in even morbidly obese *Biggest Loser* patients, Bod Pod body-fat percentages typically came very close to the iDEXA body-fat percentages (on average 1 to 2 percentage points higher). Bod Pod testing sites can now be found in most parts of the United States (1–800–4BODPOD, for Bod Pod test sites near you).

4. Bioimpedance Spectroscopy (BIS) is a promising, relatively inexpensive technology capable of not only accurately predicting body fat but also partitioning a person's lean tissue into its water and solid (muscle, organ, and bone) compartments. Sticky pads are placed on a hand and foot and then the BIS device runs an electrical current (too little to notice) through the body at multiple high and low frequencies with the impedance (opposition to electrical flow) measured. Impedance is highest in fat,

intermediate in fluid inside cells, and lowest in fluid outside of cells. With the help of Dr. Jim Matthie, a pioneer of the BIS method, my laboratory has corrected mathematical assumptions that in the past led to errant results in obese patients; now we get BIS body-fat percentages in obese and morbidly obese patients within several percent of iDEXA—plus a wealth of information on hydration.

Water changes are vital! Athletes need just the right amount of water for peak performance and new studies indicate increased water in muscle cells sends an anabolic (growth) signal. During *The Biggest Loser* show, to gain an advantage, contestants would attempt to dehydrate some weeks, load on salt and water pre-weigh-in other weeks (when they knew they won immunity from being voted off the show). Weights could swing by 20 or more pounds in one week! BIS measurements identified whether weight loss (or gain) was from fat, muscle, or water stores. Our testing of BIS will continue; stay abreast of continuing advances at www.thewowrx.com.

Other less-desirable options for determining your lean/fat percentages include:

- Body Impedance Analysis (BIA). Never confuse the much-hyped BIA scales with the BIS device discussed previously. Because BIA devices employ only limited fixed frequencies, this technique cannot offer accurate information across patient populations.

    In fact, in my experience, the most common consumer device (a stand-up BIA bathroom scale) was inaccurate: the fat percentages were all over the map, from reasonably accurate to miles off. For the extra-large *Biggest Loser* participants, despite the claims of the manufacturers, BIA scales did not work at all, often just flashing the word "error."

    BIA doesn't do well on the opposite end of the fitness spectrum either. Recently, several of my muscular ex-National Football League patients attended a supposedly state-of-the-art health screening and received body-fat percentages calculated by this gimmicky BIA technology; they were told that their body-fat percentages were over 25 percent—that's high—indicating a fat problem! When these ex-players were then tested in my office using gold standard body-composition machines, their body-fat percentages were 12 to 13 percent—in the perfectly healthy range!

- Subcutaneous fat—whether monitored via calipers or newfangled ultrasound probes—is a misleading indicator of body-fat percentage in obese folks. Stretched-out skin (especially on the upper back) and irregular stomach fat rolls (if the caliper jaws are big enough) make it difficult to obtain reproducible skin-thickness measurements. Furthermore, obese over-the-belt bellies and flabby extremities have a disproportionate amount of fat marbled deep inside, resulting in greatly underestimated body-fat percentages. For *The Biggest Loser* participants, caliper techniques underestimated body fat by 15 pounds for women to more than 25 pounds for men. Curiously, for the participants who most successfully shed fat, skin caliper measurements now overestimated body fat.

- The Mufflin equation. Many people are familiar with this method touted on various Internet weight-loss sites for calculating your resting metabolic rate by using your weight, height, age, and sex. If you work backward, assuming, as most researchers do, that lean tissue accounts for nearly all of the resting metabolic activity, then this equation also gives an estimate of your fat stores. Unfortunately, it's not very accurate. It consistently underestimated the body fat of *Biggest Loser* contestants by more than 25 pounds!

In order to calculate accurate body-fat percentages (BF percent) of *The Biggest Loser* contestants (and my own patients), I use around $200,000 worth of 21st-century gadgets and $500 of standard stuff: iDEXA ($150,000), Bod Pod ($40,000), Fitmate Resting Metabolic Rate ($8,000), BIS impedance ($5,000), calibrated big-person scale accurate to 500 pounds ($400), skin calipers ($50), and tape measure ($5).

Unfortunately, not many physicians have access to this array of technology, but they should, at least, be using the low-tech stuff! When I requested that each of the 36 *Biggest Loser* home participants get an official certified weight, few of those who weighed over 350 pounds had a doctor with a big-person calibrated scale! And none of their doctors performed waist and hip measurements, perhaps the most legitimate "free" fat test.

Step 5: Calculate Your Resting Daily Energy Expenditure (RDEE)

After you have determined your fat/lean body weight (preferably via an accurate DEXA or Bod Pod), you can now estimate your resting daily energy expenditure (RDEE) or resting metabolic rate, the number of calories your body would use if you relaxed in bed all day and night. There's some math involved: Multiply your lean tissue (in pounds) times 9.8, then, add 370 to get your RDEE (in calories per day). The equation is:

$$\text{RDEE (cal/day)} = [(100 - BF\%) \div 100] \times [\text{current weight (lbs)} \times 9.8] + 370$$

If your RDEE is based on the Mufflin equation or skin calipers, be aware that your RDEE—and your daily calorie allotment that you will calculate next—will probably be on the high side.

You can roughly estimate your RDEE based on the Mufflin equation; the formula (weight in kg, height in cm) for women is (10 × weight) plus (6.25 × height) minus (5 × age) minus 161. For men it's (10 × weight) plus (6.25 × height) minus (5 × age) plus 5. When most doctors and do-it-yourself Internet weight loss sites magically arrive at your daily calorie needs, this is usually the source. In Figures 6.1 and 6.2 (one for women, the other for men), each square represents the resting energy needs of *Biggest Loser* participants calculated at the beginning of The WOW! ℞ using this commonly used Mufflin equation. What the figures illustrate

58

HOW A PATIENT CALCULATED HER RDEE

The patient—a former volleyball player, mother of two, 5' 6" tall, and weighing 200 pounds—got an accurate body-fat percentage measurement of 46 percent.

To calculate her lean mass in pounds by using this fat percentage, she subtracted 46 percent from 100 percent to get her lean percentage: 54 percent (or 0.54).

Her lean mass in pounds is her weight (200 pounds) multiplied by her lean percentage (0.54), or 108 pounds of lean. Therefore, her body consists of 92 pounds of fat and 108 pounds of lean tissue.

Her calculated RDEE is her lean tissue (in pounds) times 9.8 plus 370. So her RDEE =108 x 9.8 + 370 = 1428 calories per day.

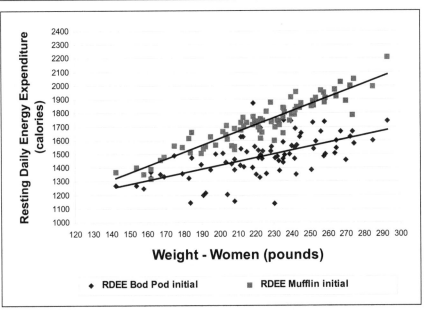

Figure 5.1 Estimated RDEE in *Biggest Loser* women based on either lean weight from Bod Pod (diamonds) or the Mufflin Equation (squares)

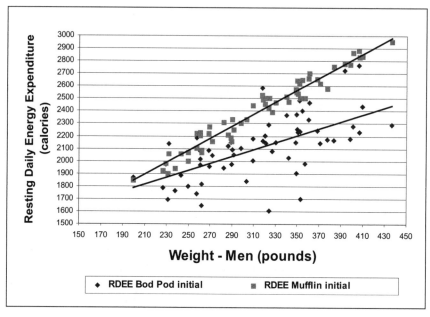

Figure 5.2 Estimated RDEE in *Biggest Loser* men based on either lean weight from Bod Pod (diamonds) or the Mufflin Equation (squares)

is that the fatter you are, the less correct the Mufflin equation becomes (i.e., the greater the difference between the Mufflin RDEE estimate and the Bod Pod RDEE estimate). These figures illustrate why accurate individualized body-fat percentage analysis is important in selecting an appropriate daily calorie allotment.

You can also estimate your RDEE based on those of *The Biggest Loser* contestants. Again, having accurate, personalized information about your own body metabolism is best, but if these technologies are not available where you live, Tables 5.1 and 5.2, gleaned from *The Biggest Loser* participants, may give obviously obese individuals a better starting point than the currently available Mufflin equation.

As you can see from the actual data points in Tables 5.1 and 5.2, huge individual variations are the norm. Individuals with more muscle are at the upper end of the RDEE range. However, in this group, I couldn't

Table 5.1. Women with Fat Rolls
(Age range: 20 to 50. Height range: 62 to 69 inches)

Weight (lbs)	Mufflin Averages RDEE (calories)	*Biggest Loser* Averages RDEE (calories) range
160	1,420	1,250–1,450
170	1,470	1,250–1,470
180	1,525	1,260–1,480
190	1,575	1,270–1,500
200	1,630	1,280–1,510
210	1,680	1,290–1,530
220	1,730	1,290–1,540
230	1,785	1,300–1,560
240	1,840	1,310–1,570
250	1,890	1,310–1,590
260	1,940	1,320–1,600
270	1,995	1,330–1,620
280	2,045	1,340–1,630

predict muscular-athletic types by their high school sports histories. Many of the more muscular participants had never participated in sports or organized exercise of any sort; conversely, some of those who earned a letter(s) in high school varsity sports were not particularly muscular and, therefore, didn't have a particularly high RDEE.

Step 6: Calculate Your Individual WOW! ℞ Nutrition Plan Daily Calorie Allotment

To determine your individual calorie allotment for The WOW! ℞, multiply your RDEE, which you've calculated previously, by 0.8. This is the least amount of calories you should take in—assuming you've been cleared by your doctor to embark on The WOW! ℞—in order to lose about 0.5 percent of your weight each week. (The exercise component we'll discuss

Table 5.2. Men with Fat Rolls
(Age range: 20 to 50. Height range: 66 to 75 inches)

Weight (lbs)	Mufflin Averages RDEE (calories)	*Biggest Loser* Averages RDEE (calories) range
230	1,980	1,730–2,120
240	2,030	1,740–2,150
250	2,080	1,750–2,040
260	2,125	1,770–2,055
270	2,170	1,780–2,070
280	2,220	1,795–2,090
300	2,315	1,825–2,120
310	2,365	1,840–2,135
320	2,410	1,855–2,150
330	2,460	1,870–2,170
340	2,505	1,880–2,185
350	2,555	1,900–2,200
360	2,600	1,910–2,215
370	2,650	1,925–2,230
380	2,695	1,940–2,250
390	2,745	1,955–2,265
400	2,790	1,970–2,280
410	2,840	1,980–2,300

later will burn off an additional 1 percent of your weight each week for the first two months, and assure that all of the weight lost is fat.)

Although calculating optimal food amounts for overweight adult exercisers to consume can be tricky, it's also important. Your body goes into starvation mode when you eat too few calories, paradoxically, lowering the amount of fat you burn. Low-carb diets make fat-burning exercise difficult because a proper fire needs kindling (carbs) to get the logs (your body fat) to burn; your body may cannibalize its own muscle for fuel when you eat too little carbohydrates and/or protein. Plus, the food you eat needs to have enough calories to minimize medical problems, such as gallstones, constipation, and electrolyte depletion, while keeping hunger at bay. During the initial seasons of *The Biggest Loser*, I kept track of the contestants' calorie intake, exercise, and weekly weight loss, and finally settled on four-fifths (80 percent) of the body's resting calorie needs (RDEE) as the mandated calorie floor. This number seemed to facilitate the most rapid fat loss while still keeping participants from being hungry and allowing them to exercise vigorously. So your calorie floor equals your RDEE multiplied by 0.8.

Using the example of the same 200-pound woman above, we multiplied her RDEE of 1,426 by 0.8 and arrived at a daily calorie allotment of 1,140, but we rounded her individualized daily calorie allotment up to 1,150. Since fat tissue also requires a teensy bit of energy to meet its resting daily energy expenditure, one could add a fudge factor amounting to a few extra daily calories for those with huge amounts of extra fat. However, for *The Biggest Loser* participants, I chose not to make any adjustments that had anything to do with fudge.

The truth is, most doctors, dietitians, trainers, and street-corner fitness gurus who counsel the obese on weight loss either pull the desired daily calorie intake out of a hat or rely on simple, but inaccurate, measures like BMI (weight (lbs) $\times$ 703 $\div$ height (in)^2). Women are typically given the nice round numbers of 1,200, 1,000, or 900 calories per day; large men are typically assigned 2,100, 1,800, or 1,500 calories. Problem is, for a stocky 5' 8" ex-jock mom, the above standard is far too low, heightening chances of hunger, muscle loss, and rebound appetite surges; for a relatively normal-appearing 5' 7" nonathletic woman with "iceberg" obesity (a seemingly normal weight and BMI, but with high fat levels and low amounts of muscle), the reverse will be true, perhaps slowing down fat loss and sidestepping the positive reinforcement of rapid results.

Fortunately, *The Biggest Loser* home participants who stuck with their personalized calorie allotments experienced little or no hunger and were able to safely fuel moderate to vigorous 60-minute morning and evening workouts.

Step 7: Calculate Your WOW! Weight

Your WOW! weight—your "ideal" weight without dangerous levels of abdominal fat—equals your original lean weight plus an "ideal" amount of fat, 20–27 percent for women, 12–20 percent for men. So, women, your WOW! weight will be roughly 75 percent lean plus 25 percent fat; men, your WOW! weight will be roughly 85 percent lean plus 15 percent fat. (For this calculation, we'll ignore the fact that on The WOW! ℞, the lean tissue is "changing"; you're naturally losing water that "services" fat while gaining muscle and fluids associated with being physically fit.)

Here's the formula:

WOW! weight equals lean weight divided by the percent lean you are aiming for. We've said 75 percent lean, 25 percent fat is an ideal woman's composition. So, using the example of the 200-pound woman above: WOW! weight = 108 pounds (original lean) ÷ 0.75 = 144 pounds. Therefore, her WOW! goal weight would be 144 pounds (by the way, a woman who is 5′ 6″ tall with 108 pounds of lean tissue is quite athletic).

Step 8: Purchase Inexpensive Home Gym Equipment

See the details in Push/Pull/Twist Training—Chapter Eight.

Step 9: Start The WOW! ℞ and Begin Losing Fat!

Chapter Six

Understanding Healthy Eating for Fat Loss

THE WOW! ℞ NUTRITIONAL PLAN

The healthy eating plan for The WOW! ℞ emphasizes eating lean protein, nonfat dairy products (or calcium-fortified soy substitutes), lots of high-fiber fruits and vegetables, and whole grains (in moderation please!). It emphasizes the good you must eat, not the bad I'd like you to avoid. My experience from the home participants, however, reinforces my belief that in order to get dramatic fat-loss results, you should initially learn to count calories and compulsively write down everything that passes your lips (in a notebook or on an Excel spreadsheet), then tally your total caloric intake nightly. Make sure you consume at least enough to match your caloric allotment! Split your calories up into three meals and several snacks or post-exercise anabolic shakes. Don't skip meals; this may paradoxically result in an increased caloric intake and a blunted ability to exercise off calories. Although not etched in stone, I'm aiming for an intake of approximately 30 to 35 percent protein, 40 to 45 percent carbohydrate, and 20 to 30 percent fat. These percentages seem to handle satiety while providing enough carbohydrates and protein for dramatic fat loss with conservation or growth of muscle. Finally, after two weeks of going it on your own, provide your dietitian with one complete representative three-day summary at the beginning of your third week to make sure you're mastering calorie counting. Even if you're a calorie-counting Einstein, it would still behoove you to discuss the fine points of food shopping, advance planning and preparation of meals, and navigating fat-filled restaurant menus. As an alternative (if you are unable to find or afford a dietitian), you can plug in the foods on a Web site such as www.fitday.com or http://nat.crgq.com/mainnat.html, which will calculate your total calories as well as the macronutrient percentages (i.e., fat versus carbohydrate versus protein) and micronutrient quantities (i.e., minerals and antioxidants).

Depending on your calculated individualized calorie allotment, your "core" foods (what you should eat every day) will differ slightly. The following daily consumption requirements are approximated; your actual calorie count will ensure that you are not consuming too many—or too few—calories. Again, it bears repeating, eating fewer calories per day than are suggested, or God only knows, taking another diet pill are shortcuts to sickness, not health.

At a minimum, consume the following "core" foods:

- If your daily calorie allotment is 1,000 to 1,249 calories, you should consume:

   2 lean protein servings (4 ounces raw, 3 ounces cooked)

   2 nonfat or low-fat dairy product servings (8 ounces)

   2 whole-grain/high-fiber carbohydrate servings ($^1/_2$ cup)

   2 fruit servings (size of average apple)

   6 or more vegetable servings (1 cup raw, $^1/_2$ cup cooked)

   6 to 8 glasses water (8 ounces each)

- If your daily calorie allotment is 1,250 to 1,499 calories, you should consume:

   3 servings lean protein

   2 to 3 servings nonfat or low-fat dairy products

   2 servings whole-grain/high-fiber carbohydrates

   2 to 3 fruit servings

   6 or more vegetable servings

   6 to 8 glasses water

- If your daily calorie allotment is 1,500-plus calories, you should consume:

  4 servings lean protein

  3 servings nonfat or low-fat dairy products

  3 servings whole-grain/high-fiber carbohydrates

  3 fruit servings

  7 or more vegetable servings

  6 to 8 glasses water

Ideally, you should eat five to six times a day (breakfast, lunch, dinner, plus two to three snacks or anabolic shakes—more on these later), and each meal or snack should contain both a protein source and a carbohydrate source. By breaking up your calories into five to six meals per day, you will minimize hunger and maximize the amount of available calories for your body to burn in order to digest your food. The Nutrition Plan (Section Three) of this book provides examples of serving sizes and calorie counts of lean protein, dairy products/substitutes, whole-grain/high-fiber carbohydrates, fruits and vegetables, as well as sample daily menus for various calorie allotments.

If you have extra calories left over after eating all of the above core nutrition foods, you can add any additional food from the preceding categories, or may add other wholesome grains or an extra serving of heathful unsaturated fats, such as olive oil, avocados, olives, tree nuts (almonds, walnuts, pecans), flaxseed oil, or unsweetened cocoa powder.

You may also benefit from taking a daily multivitamin supplement. Week 14 of the Week-by-Week portion (Section Two) of this book contains all the information you need to know about vitamin supplements, however, discuss your individual needs with your physician or dietitian.

How Do You Stick to Your Calorie Guidelines?

Sorry. You must count calories. And to do that you've got to accurately measure food using a food scale, as well as measuring cups and spoons. (Read all about calorie counting in the Nutrition Plan, Section Three.) God knows, we've all looked for shortcuts—eating only "healthful" foods, eating only when you're hungry, eating small protein-carb snacks every three hours, eating only before six in the evening, limiting portion sizes, even paying a food delivery service to cater meals with supposedly the proper calorie counts and protein-to-fat-to-carb ratios. If you stick with low-calorie delivery service fare, you will lose weight. Problem is, since you haven't learned much, if anything, about nutrition (and most weight-loss plans teach you nothing about exercise), you don't have a prayer of a chance at keeping weight off in the long run.

In the past, many *Biggest Loser* contestants elected to wing it; they figured they'd just do the right thing: Eat small portion sizes of lean meat and fresh fruits and vegetables when they were hungry. In fact, during the first two regular seasons of the show, non-calorie-counting *Biggest Loser* participants did great; they lost 16 percent of their original weights! However, their accomplishments were overshadowed by the calorie-counting contestants, who lost almost 27 percent of their original weights, nearly twice as much!

True, that statistic is clouded because the calorie counters also tended to work out harder and longer—they were generally more serious about all aspects of the plan. Also true, calorie counting is a giant pain in the you-know-what, but there's something very powerful about writing down exactly what you eat and learning the caloric value of every morsel that touches your tongue. Those black-and-white entries attack mindless eating and force accountability. So keep a food journal; jot down every calorie for every food every day. Be anal retentive for at least the entire first four months. You'll be shocked by how much you learn about food—and yourself.

Counting calories is no cakewalk. It takes time to write down the exact details of what you've eaten after each meal. It takes time to tally up your totals at the end of each day. It takes a calorie-counting book, an inexpensive kitchen food scale, and at least a few dietary consultations. A registered dietitian (RD) can supervise your calorie-counting education, making sure you choose the right kinds of foods, journal in proper portion sizes, decipher hidden ingredients in cooked foods, and account for different cooking techniques—even professional chefs and other food whizzes benefit. For instance, roasting or grilling (using dry heat to cook) will remove water, while steaming may add water to high-liquid-content fresh fruit, vegetables, and lean protein. So 3 ounces of steamed/stewed chicken breast is 129 calories and 2.6 grams of fat, but when roasted it's 140 calories, 3 grams of fat—more water is removed with roasting, as opposed to steaming, increasing the calorie density.

You can explore Internet sites that will help you start food journals and shoulder the calculation grunt work for you—especially protein versus fat versus carb breakdowns and assessments of calcium and antioxidant adequacy. The question is: Do Web sites that automatically compute caloric values of what you eat (or are considering eating) foster retention and long-term learning or do they become crutches? The eventual goal is for you to "instinctively" estimate calories. So I suggest you spend at least part of the time with a calorie-counting manual, slugging through the numbers by hand.

Once you've mastered basic calorie counting, you can start deciphering labels, figuring out sugar, fat, and micronutrient amounts, and sniffing out toxins like trans fats, nitrites, and mercury. Bingo, you've taken the first step to becoming a certified food expert! And that's a lifesaving skill.

Exactly What Types of Food Do You Eat?

Carbohydrates

- Depending on your individual calorie allotment, you should eat two to three fresh (not dried) fruit servings per day; otherwise you may need a daily multivitamin. No juice—toss out your juicers, not your food's valuable fiber! A whole orange will fill you up much more than 4 ounces of orange juice!

- Eat six or more vegetable servings per day; otherwise you may need a daily multivitamin. Try to eat various different-colored vegetables each day to increase the variety of vitamins, minerals, and phytochemicals (antioxidents) that you're eating—light and dark green, purple, red, yellow, and orange vegetables all have different valuable nutrient profiles. Yes, sweet potatoes and winter squash are starchier and more calorie dense than other vegetables but in moderation are still fine (without the toppings!).

- Whole grains in moderation: Beans, barley, brown rice, whole wheat, couscous, millet, oat bran; products such as sprouted grain Ezekiel bread, Wasa crackers, Kashi GoLean cereal, and whole-grain tortillas, to name a few options. There's a ton of confusion with the "whole-" grain moniker. It means minimally processed grain, i.e., the fiber-rich outer kernel and the vitamin- and mineral-rich inner germ have not been removed. Advertisers try to trick us by making foods sound as if they contain whole grains when they do not. Don't be taken in by the following terms: seven grain, made with wheat flour, brown, enriched. . . look at the ingredients. First on the list of whole-grain products will be whole wheat, whole oats, whole rye, or another whole grain; ideally, one serving will contain at least 3 grams of fiber.

- No caloric fluids, except skim milk and soymilk, are to be consumed. That's correct, no fruit juice, sweetened teas, juice "drinks," lemonade, or sodas. . . the body has a difficult time registering the calories consumed in liquid form—you will not feel full after drinking a soda, but you will feel full after eating a high-fiber tortilla.

- No beer, wine, or "hard" liquor. While alcoholic beverages in moderation have health benefits for those without the "addiction" gene, they're not only a stiff slug of hard-to-register liquid calories, they're also appetite enhancers!

- There's always an exception to every rule, right? You'll be excited to learn that the no-simple-sugar/no-caloric-fluids rules change during the immediate post-exercise period—and for good reason—post-workout anabolic shakes build muscle. . . more to follow!

Lean Protein

- Red meat should be kept to a minimum (one serving per week) because it is higher in saturated fat than other protein sources. Very lean red meat (like sirloin or tri-tip steak) is okay occasionally, but the leaner the beef, the tougher it is, therefore, most people prefer the taste and texture of the higher-fat cuts. So you may choose to eliminate red meat altogether in favor of skinless turkey, chicken, and fish. As a general rule, menstruating women who ingest no red meat should consult a dietitian for vegetarian alternatives or consider taking an iron and B supplement.
- Eggs: Egg whites (or egg substitute) are essentially pure protein and are preferred, but a whole egg a day is okay to eat, too. It turns out that the amount of cholesterol contained in an egg yolk is not enough to induce heart disease when you're eating a healthful diet like this one.
- Fish: Depending on your individual calorie allotment, you should eat at least two to four fresh fish servings per week; adolescents and women of child-bearing age should stick to low-mercury varieties, such as salmon, small shellfish (not lobster, which is higher in mercury), cod, and flounder, with only one serving per week of moderate mercury-containing varieties such as tuna—high levels of mercury have been shown to affect the growing nervous system in developing babies and young people. When in doubt, have your doctor check your blood mercury levels.

  Fish with the highest levels of mercury—including swordfish, shark, mackerel, king, and tilefish—contain up to nine times as much mercury as low-mercury fish and should be avoided. One serving a week of these fish is probably safe for adult men and women past child-bearing age, but I'd prefer you obtain heart-attack-preventing fish fat by ingesting multiple servings of low- and moderate-mercury-containing varieties.

- Vegetarians: Beans and legumes (such as black beans, chickpeas, edamame or soybeans, kidney beans, lentils, lima beans, navy beans, pinto beans, split peas, white beans) are high in carbohydrates but also contain a good amount of protein; miso, soybeans, soy burgers, and tofu are also a good vegan or vegetarian source of protein.

Healthy Fats

Monounsaturated and polyunsaturated fats (including omega-3 and omega-6 fatty acids) are the newly crowned "good fats" that actually lower cholesterol and prevent heart disease. While we recommend minimizing all fat in general because of its high calorie content, these heart-healthy fats (almonds, pecans, walnuts, olive oil, canola oil, flaxseed oil or ground flaxseeds, avocados, and, of course, the fat contained in fish) are good for you in small doses.

The "bad fats"—saturated fat and trans fats—have been shown to increase the risk of heart disease and strokes. Foods that are high in saturated fat and/or transfats include whole and 2 percent milk, cream, butter, cheese, lard, red meat, coconut oil, palm kernel oil, and all foods with hydrogenated or partially hydrogenated ingredients (read the label!), including margarine, shortening, commercially deep-fried foods, and many processed foods, such as candy bars and potato chips. Avoid these foods!

Fresh and Dried Herbs and Spices

The sky's the limit. Try basil, cilantro, oregano, parsley, thyme, rosemary, dill, cinnamon, ginger, cloves, Italian seasonings blend, vanilla extract, garlic, ginger, mustard, horseradish, and vinegar.

Will Eating All-Protein for the First Few Weeks Jump-Start Your Fat Loss?

Three things: Number one, it's physically impossible to go all-protein. I'll never forget an interview I had with one of the prospective trainers for the initial *Biggest Loser*. She claimed to get amazing results from starting off her clients on an 80 percent protein diet! But what she didn't know was that this was almost impossible to achieve—most foods that we think of as "protein" actually also contain carbs, water, and fat. I knew that, for more than one meal, achieving 80 percent protein is impossible. As you can see in Table 6.1, with the exception of skinless roasted turkey breast, canned tuna packed in water, and egg whites, no "protein" food even has 80 percent protein in it! Even protein powders mixed in water have less than 65 percent of their calories from protein!

I broke down her "all-protein" diet: Her clients were taking in around 35 percent of their calories as protein, with relatively high fat levels. She was off by a whopping 45 percent!

Which brings me to point number two: Although the generally accepted opinion is that mono- and polyunsaturated fats do not cause heart disease—except nonspecifically via high-calorie levels leading to waistline weight gain—it's best to systematically avoid high-saturated fat foods. By the way, for all of you who are faddishly chomping on higher-fat snacks such as almonds, or licking spoonfuls of peanut butter for your afternoon snack, please note that certain whole-grain products and even some fruits, because of their higher water, fiber, and protein content, may be much more satiating (per calorie consumed)! And nuts and nut butters are mostly fat—for example, look at Table 6.1—peanut butter is only 16 percent protein (even whole oats are higher!).

Point number three: Yes, most, if not all, of the extra quick weight

Table 6.1 Protein Foods

FOODS	Calories	Protein (%)	Fat (%)	Sat Fat (%)	Mono (%)	Poly (%)	Carbs (%)	Fiber
Poultry								
Turkey (white, roasted, no skin), 3 oz	131	80	20	6	3	5	0	negligible
Chicken (white, roasted, no skin), 3 oz	137	79	21	6	7	4	0	negligible
Turkey (dark, roasted, no skin), 3 oz	156	64	36	12	8	11	0	negligible
Chicken (dark, roasted, no skin), 3 oz	159	59	41	11	15	10	0	negligible
Fish								
Tuna, canned, water packed, 3 oz	99	93	7	2	1	3	0	negligible
Shrimp, baked or broiled, 3 oz	130	66	31	6	11	10	3	negligible
Salmon, broiled, 3 oz	98	58	41	7	15	14	1	negligible
Vegetarian								
Soyburger, cooked, 3 oz	162	47	45	7	11	24	8	4 grams
Dairy								
Egg white (1 large)	18	91	0	0	0	0	9	negligible
Plain nonfat yogurt	137	41	3	2	1	0	56	negligible
Skim (nonfat) milk	86	39	5	3	1	0	56	negligible
Chocolate skim milk	168	20	4	2	1	0	76	negligible
1% milk, 8 oz	102	31	23	14	7	1	46	negligible
Egg whole (1 large)	77	33	64	24	24	8	3	negligible
Mozzarella cheese (4⅝ in. long)	78	40	56	35	16	2	4	negligible

Table 6.1 Protein Foods, *continued*

FOODS	Calories	Protein (%)	Fat (%)	Sat Fat (%)	Mono (%)	Poly (%)	Carbs (%)	Fiber
Beef								
Pork, cooked, 3 oz, lean only	114	57	43	15	19	3	0	negligible
Beef tenderloin, separable lean only	175	57	43	16	16	2	0	negligible
Ground beef, extra lean, cooked, 3 oz	213	41	59	23	26	2	0	negligible
Nuts								
Almonds (12)	83	15	80	6	51	19	6	negligible
Peanut butter, 1 tbs	95	16	75	15	36	20	9	negligible

"Carb" Foods	Calories	Protein (%)	Fat (%)	Sat Fat (%)	Mono (%)	Poly (%)	Carbs (%)	Fiber
Fruit								
Strawberries, 1 cup, raw	43	10	14	1	2	7	77	3 grams
Orange, raw, one large	85	9	3	0	0	1	89	4 grams
Grains								
Oats, raw, ⅓ cup	104	18	16	3	5	6	65	3 grams
Kashi GoLean cereal (½ cup)	70	37	7	0			56	5 grams
Kashi GoLean Crunch cereal (½ cup)	95	19	13	0			59	4 grams

loss associated with high-protein (low-carb) diets is a result of lost lean tissue (mostly glycogen and water)—certainly nothing to brag about. Conversely, there have been several studies that indicate a 30 percent protein diet results in better retention of lean mass and more fat loss.

So, to answer your question: yes, if you go "all-protein" (very low carb) for a few weeks, you will drop more weight—but not more fat. And the extra water/glycogen weight that you lose will come right back as soon as you incorporate carbs into your diet again. The bottom line: it's not worth it.

Do the Carbs in Fruits and Grains Cause Obesity?

In a word, no. Recently, 49,000 post-menopausal women, who lowered their fat intake and increased their carbs, were studied over an eight-year time span. The results: They did not gain weight as predicted by Atkins advocates and other disciples of the low-carb religion. Want further verification? *The Biggest Loser* home contestants lost far more weight than any other documented home-based weight-loss group, while consuming a diet high in complex carbohydrates, namely fruits and vegetables.

What Should You Avoid?

Avoid processed foods, sugars, simple carbohydrates (such as white rice, white pasta, white bread), saturated fats (such as butter, full-fat cheeses, red meat, dark-meat poultry), trans fats (such as margarine, fast foods, and foods containing hydrogenated or partially hydrogenated oils), and try to detox off artificial fats and sweeteners. Simple carbs and sugar found in processed, nutrient-poor, calorie-dense, or fake foods are sometimes referred to as high-glycemic-index foods (blood-sugar-spiking foods). Diets packed with high-glycemic-index foods have clearly been linked to diabetes and heart disease; some healthy foods though, specifically, sweet potatoes, carrots, watermelon, and even nonfat Lactaid milk, are high glycemic, but not problematic to your health. Why? Despite the simple structure of these natural nonprocessed carbs allowing rapid enzymatic conversion to sugar by the body, they are lower-calorie items, and you would have to literally ingest pounds of these foods for a negative impact. So for practical purposes, there's little to fear.

Sodas warrant a special caution. The body's appetite-control center has difficulty registering liquid calories, in part explaining why the average American mainlines nearly 150 pounds of sugar each year—mostly via sweet drinks. Diet sodas (and other foods that are artificially sweetened) may have few or zero calories, but the sweet taste still leads to a higher insulin spike in your bloodstream and may keep you craving real sweets. In fact, switching from regular soda to artificially sweetened soda has never been shown to lead to weight loss! Similarly, no one knows whether fat-reduced chips will keep your taste buds habituated and set the stage for eventual relapse with "real" high-fat foods. In my opinion, the better part of valor is to stay away. The same goes for energy bars, meal replacements, and other "health foods" often marketed by means of photos of people with muscular builds on the packaging. Although most of us understand that red meat contains saturated fat and other potentially harmful substances, few realize that many of these so-called health or sports-bars have far less than optimal protein sources, while containing hidden saturated fats and trace trans fats. As a general principle, it's buyer beware.

Allow me one brief digression. From an energy standpoint, 500 calories of skinless white turkey meat with broccoli and a salad with vinaigrette dressing are just as fattening as 500 calories of Häagen-Daz French Vanilla ice cream topped with real whipped cream. Here's the catch. We typically eat the same weight of food per day, and the ice cream has far more calories per ounce than the lean protein, vegetable, and good fat meal.

Additionally, lean protein and high-fiber foods have special satiation powers, making you feel full more quickly and for a longer period of time. Lastly, the body has to expend a lot more calories to digest protein and fiber than it does to digest fat and sugar. So, although a 500-calorie healthy meal and a 500-calorie ice cream dessert are, on the surface, "equally fattening," as you can see, even moderate junk food intakes can quickly translate into unflattering flab.

Will Quitting Cigarettes Make You Eat More?

With no exercise, probably yes. However, one of the true great offshoots of The WOW! ℞ was keeping over half of the smokers cigarette free at two years. But the real shocker was that they lost weight as effectively as their nonsmoking brethren. There goes the "I refuse to stop smoking 'cause I'll gain weight" argument!

Is There a Downside to Healthful Low-Fat, Low-Sugar, and High-Antioxidant Foods?

There are two prickly problems with healthful, lifesaving foods—time and money. Fast food is "quick and easy" compared with shopping for, and then preparing, fresh fruit, vegetables, and lean protein several times a week. And few people discuss the glaring fact that, calorie for calorie, the healthful satiating foods we're touting are more expensive than sugar and fat. In order to contain the obesity epidemic, these economic issues need to be addressed.

The time factor can be circumvented with convenience items, such as pre-washed, pre-cut fruits and veggies, canned tuna and white meat chicken, soy protein patties, and a George Foreman grill for easy-on-the-pocket grilled chicken. Cost factors can be partially allayed with frozen fruits and vegetables, together with stockpiling seasonal items. Even then, in the short term, fresh fruit, vegetables, and lean protein will set you back a few extra bucks, but these extra costs will be the best investment you'll ever make. A recent UCLA/Rand study showed that obesity increases a person's annual health-care costs by 40 percent and medication costs by 80 percent! And obesity kills! You can't put a price tag on life.

How Do You Prevent Hunger?

To eat or not to eat—in a thousand tongues the stomach talks to the brain and the brain talks to the stomach. Recently discovered neurointestinal languages include insulin, melanocortin, neuropeptide Y, PYY, thyroxine, leptin, cholecystokinin, and ghrelin, to name a few. Don't worry; you don't need to memorize these. Suffice to say, we have miles left to travel on our journey to translate the chemical basis for hunger and how to manipulate it safely with drugs. For now, regular exercise and an organized healthful dietary approach, eating foods with fiber and protein with each meal and snack, preferably at the same time each day and not skipping meals, can work wonders! It may seem logical that if you can power past a meal or two, you're eating fewer calories and are therefore on your way to that "thin" wardrobe buried in the back of the closet. But the preponderance of evidence is closer to this: Skip a meal, risk a binge. Studies show that calories saved by meal abstinence are usually made up for (and then some) when you finally do decide to eat what often turns out to be a whopper of a meal.

As noted, both fiber and protein foods possess special satiation properties. Your best bet for ultimate fat loss is to stick with high-fiber whole fruit, vegetables, and whole grains (in moderation) together with lean protein.

What If, Despite All This, You're Still Hungry?

Eat. Remember, even state-of-the-art scientific determinations of your true caloric needs may be off by hundreds of calories. Be sure to select extra snacks with the most bang for the caloric buck. A salad with a pop of protein—translation: 2 to 3 ounces of skinless chicken—or a slice of whole grain bread with a stab of tuna, a boiled egg, half a fruit and nonfat cottage cheese, yogurt, or soy milk. . . yes, even a small handful of tree nuts on occasion. . .you get the picture. Lastly, when you're hungry, make a point of letting everything hang out in your thought journal. If you recognize that you actually are more upset, exhausted, or stressed than truly hungry, get your psychologist coach involved. Don't penny-pinch, don't deny, and don't delay.

Fortunately, consistent hunger occurred in less than one in five *Biggest Loser* contestants, and they were told to gradually increase their daily caloric allowances by 50 to 100 calories for several days, and then reevaluate their food urges. Fast-food binges and chocolate cravings were the subject of a host of longingly described daydreams, but to my knowledge, they were acted upon less than a handful of times—and then mostly with dire consequences. You see, once you detox off of ice cream and cookies, several (initially delicious) bites can turn the bowels inside out with pain and diarrhea. We've all been there.

The wacky truth? The bigger problem is more often the opposite: "It's just too much food, Doc! I can't stuff down all the calories you want!" Under those conditions, I recommend goosing the salads with more good fats like avocado and olive oil dressing and sneaking in starchy vegetables.

Are There Better Times of the Day to Eat?

Yes. Food timing is one of the secret WOW! ℞ ingredients. The short- and long-term success of the WOW! ℞ depends, in part, on techniques borrowed from sports medicine that exploit the body's 24-hour circadian rhythm and unique time-dependent nutritional opportunities post-exercise.

First off, adhering to a day-in, day-out eating and workout pattern aligns the body's physiologic functions and psychological well-being, thereby reinforcing exercise and diet compliance while enhancing exercise effort and calorie burn. Believe me, most people notice improvements in all aspects of their lives after they're firmly entrenched in a regular daily schedule.

Secondly, we can boost the dual calorie-burning and muscle-retention properties of exercise during planned weight loss by drinking a readily digestible liquid protein-carbohydrate cocktail within 30 minutes of a strenuous workout. For our purposes, this maneuver is doubly effective; it puts your WOW! ℞ calorie allotment to best use by protecting muscle and by aiding your body's ability to burn body fat.

What Is an Instantly Digestible Protein-Carb Cocktail?

That's just scientific code for a whey protein simple-carbohydrate drink!

Simple Carbs are Sugars. Simple Carbs are High-Glycemic Public Enemies! They Should Be Sworn Off for Life, Right?

That depends. It's common knowledge that exponentially increased consumption of dietary sugar over the last 50 years directly parallels the obesity epidemic. It's also true that sugar, and all its high-glycemic kin (i.e., rapidly absorbed carbohydrates) have a nasty habit of sending blood sugar, then insulin, sky-high, thereby shuttling calories into fat cells for long-term storage. Adding insult to injury, the insulin spikes often overtreat the blood sugar, potentially retickling the appetite—and yet more junk food cravings. So, by day's end, the abdominal tire is a little more inflated.

But sugar consumed, followed by insulin surges, have schizophrenic tendencies. They can have an entirely different effect! For 30 to 45 minutes after exercise, muscle membranes light up with insulin receptors, allowing insulin, for a fleeting period of time, to switch gears and become a legal anabolic steroid!

Insulin's anabolic actions involve muscle building, muscle feeding, and muscle protection:

- Muscle building—increases transport of building-block amino acids, revs protein-building enzymes, and blocks some exercise-induced protein damage.
- Muscle feeding—pushes in glucose, facilitates storage of energy as glycogen (critical for effective exercise), and increases blood flow to carry in other nutrients and discard waste products.
- Muscle protection—insulin suppresses muscle tissues' arch enemy, cortisol, the hormone secreted in response to low blood glucose, stress, and rigorous exercise that initiates muscle breakdown.

Whey protein and simple sugars each stimulate insulin release; together they send insulin levels higher still. When this occurs in the fleeting post-exercise window—bam!—this quickly digestible duo saves the day for muscle; a switch is flipped from "exercise injury and breakdown" to "rebuilding and enlarging" muscle.

Quick refresher course: Stay away from sugar intake during any other time of the day—then it's linked to appetite disturbances, fat gain, and elevated diabetes and heart-disease risk!

How Do You Play This Sport Nutrition "Angle"?

You've got three choices:

1. Buy an energy-dense muscle-recovery drink like Endurox.
2. Get protein powder—consisting of 8 grams whey, 1 gram glutamine—at your local drugstore or health food store and mix in 30 grams (2 tablespoons) of table sugar with an antioxidant pill and a pinch of salt in 12 ounces of water. (Adding readily absorbed forms of antioxidants such as vitamin C [250 mg] and vitamin E [100 IU] offers theoretical but as yet unproved advantage.)

3. Or you can use basic foods to get a natural nutritional blast: Introducing, direct from your local grocery store, the all-natural, legal, and delicious anabolic shakes.

The secret behind these shakes is:

- Lactose-free skim milk, which has slowly absorbed lactose already broken down to simple sugars.
- Blended fruit, providing more slowly absorbed sugars.
- Antioxidants from the fruit, as adjuncts to minimizing muscle damage.
- Whey protein and glutamine are primary constituents of nonfat ricotta cheese and skim milk.

Here's my favorite color and favorite shake; the other delicious anabolic shake recipes can be found in Section Three. Enjoy!

PURPLE COW SHAKE

1/3 cup   nonfat ricotta cheese
1 cup   lactose-free nonfat milk
1/2 cup   frozen blackberries or blueberries
1/2   banana
2 tbs   frozen grape juice concentrate

Place all ingredients in the blender and blend thoroughly. Makes two servings.

Calories: 163
Protein: 11 grams
Fat: 0 grams
Carbohydrate: 30 grams

FAT-LOSS TRICKS

I don't believe in gimmicks or shortcuts, but there are a few "real" fat-loss tricks. Here's one you can have fun with: Lose calories by drinking properly timed ice water or steaming hot tea.

It takes one calorie of energy to cool down or heat up one liter of water one degree Celsius (Celsius [C] is the accepted measurement in the medical field). If you drink a liter (around a quart) jug of a piping hot noncaloric beverage (90° C), the body "loses" around 50 calories getting your body temperature back into equilibrium at its usual 37 degrees Celsius (98.6° F). Or, if you're loafing at home in front of the TV and drink a liter of iced noncaloric fluid (0° C), your body "loses" about 35 calories getting the body temperature back to baseline. Of course, the same rules apply for chilled or heated solid food. The more you force your body to work to maintain a normal body temperature, the more calories you burn!

Since we take in three to four liters or more of food and drink a day, simple temperature manipulations could burn an extra 100 calories per day, which over a year might translate to 10 pounds of fat lost. And since it's been estimated that the entire obesity epidemic is being fueled by a daily consumption of 100 excess calories, this temperature trick could, on paper anyway, save the country.

But before you run off and spread the news at the water cooler tomorrow, there are a couple of quick caveats:

- Order iced fluids/foods when you're feeling on the chilly side—obviously if you have iced fluids/foods immediately after exercise or on a hot day, you're helping the body adjust the temperature back toward normal—therefore, the body will expend *less* calories compared with room-temperature fluids! This is good for an athlete trying to conserve energy, but not so good for an obese individual trying to burn off every last drop of energy.
- Order hot items when you're feeling warm.

- A very important note: Early in an exercise program, obese folks have trouble getting rid of heat and are at risk of heat toxicity when exercising in warm weather. So for the first few months when you're out of shape, stay with room-temperature fluids during exercise.
- When it's cold outside, set the inside thermostat as cool as you can reasonably tolerate. If you want to go one step further, chew ice chips. Stay away from ice cubes—they're a cracked tooth waiting to happen.
- When it's hot outside, set the thermostat indoors as high as you can reasonably tolerate. (Are you aware that the resting energy needs of people who live in tropical climates tend to be 10 to 20 percent higher than those living in more temperate latitudes?)
- When it's cold outside, dress as lightly as you comfortably can. Of course, you can go too far, so add the next layer of clothing before your teeth start chattering.

Other Fat-Burning Tricks and Secrets

Remember that old commercial tag line: Great taste, less calories? Well, pre-exercise snacks may fit that bill. Time a protein/carb snack—perhaps a third of a cup of cereal with skim milk, or an egg and a wedge of fruit, or a glass of soy milk—immediately before a workout (if you're able to tolerate this without becoming nauseous). This trick works because exercise makes digestion far less efficient. The body has to burn up a certain amount of calories in order to physically digest the food you eat—not surprisingly, fat is easiest to absorb, protein the most difficult—so in a healthy diet roughly 15 percent of foods' calories are expended during digestion. But when you eat immediately before a workout, assimilating the nutrients temporarily becomes more difficult—depending on exercise intensity, genetics, your body-fat percentage and the type of food eaten. Inefficient digestion during exercise means up to 50 percent of foods' calories might be expended during digestion—so you get great taste, less calories.

Some have suggested you chew sugarless gum (5 calories/piece) to lose weight—I'm okay with that—gum in your mouth may discourage mindless snacking—but remember since chewing burns 11 calories per hour, you have to chomp on one piece for about 30 minutes before you begin to lose weight (60 minutes for a 10-calorie piece of regular gum). However, as previously stated, I have reservations about artificial sweeteners, and if you plan to drop 105 calories by chewing one solitary piece of Dentyne for 10 hours, you're guaranteed jaw joint pain and dental bills.

Caffeine may slightly increase the metabolic rate and augment fat burning under certain conditions, so it's an okay aid in moderation—unless you have insomnia, panic attacks, anxiety, or heart palpitations. In those cases decaffeinated coffee, tea, or plain old tap water with a slice of lemon is best.

After a snack or a meal, get out of the kitchen! Wait, wait, and wait some more before even thinking about a second helping. The brain's satiation center is a lagging indicator; it can take 20 to 30 minutes until the brain gets the stomach's "I'm full!" signal.

Don't tempt yourself. Just say no to high-fat, high-sugar, high-calorie foods in your home or office surroundings. Clean out all of your kitchen cabinets, the refrigerator, your desk drawer stashes. . . if you have to throw the food away, do it. Replace junk food with healthy snacks so that you'll always have something healthy readily available when hunger hits. Don't live in denial, communicate. Verbalize your needs to family members and coworkers—many have no idea how tempting their desktop dish of chocolate candy really is. They need to understand your fat-loss goals.

Grocery shop after you've just eaten (you tend to buy foods on impulse when you go to the store hungry), and stick to a prewritten grocery list. Substitute healthy, lifesaving foods you can learn to love for killer foods you're dying to eat.

Forget the old wives' tale that food ingested late at night is somehow metabolized differently. A calorie is a calorie regardless of the time of day it passes your lips. If you're hungry, a complex carb/lean protein snack three hours before bedtime is okay, but avoid late-night fat, caffeine, or carbonated drinks—they cause the gastroesophageal sphincter to open up, an invitation for reflux, the burning sensation behind the chest bone that's so bothersome to many obese people, especially at night when gravity no longer helps to keep the stomach contents away from the esophagus. When we're sitting up and awake, the simple act of swallowing dilutes the reflux acid; but during sleep, with no automatic swallowing, the acid lingers in the esophagus and can create local ulcers and may also escalate throat and esophageal cancer risk, as well as asthma and insomnia.

Finally, don't freak out if you succumb to an occasional splurge. Get back on the healthy eating plan as quickly as possible! Almost every single person successfully losing fat with The WOW! ℞ has admitted to falling off the wagon once in a while—the key was that they didn't beat themselves up (much) and got right back on. So an occasional lapse is a small blip in the big picture. Just don't forget how you feel the day after a splurge: Probably hung over and sick! Instead, push toward that happy feeling of fit and healthy.

Chapter Seven

Understanding Fat-Loss Exercise

THE WOW! ℞ FAT-LOSS EXERCISE PROGRAM

When it comes to body fat, Americans are in deep denial. The clothes we now buy are actually several sizes larger than what the label size says. Similarly, we've bought into "dumbed-down" exercise. Sadly, the problem starts with the advice Americans are given. Our Surgeon General recommends overweight Americans desirous of weight loss initiate exercise with a 10-minute walk three times a week, working up to 30 minutes of walking or other form of moderate activity five times a week. That measly activity? For a 200-pound person, it equates to a mere 525 extra calories of energy expended per week! Even morbidly obese sedentary Americans have far more capability than that! Yes, walking 30 minutes, five days a week has some cardiovascular health benefits, but it has no weight-loss power.

Honestly, the most you can hope for is to slow down your yearly muscle losses and fat gains. *The Biggest Loser* participants illustrate this exercise conundrum perfectly: Contestant hopefuls reported two hours (the men) to three hours (the women) of walking-equivalent exercise per week. But they still gained fistfuls of fat—specifically, they gained almost 10 pounds during the prior year! And their treadmill test results showed that they had no conditioning; only two of the first 172 participants lasted longer than an average completely sedentary person!

True fact: one morbidly obese patient told me when he used to finish his three-times-a-week, 30-minute elliptical workouts, he felt he was absolutely busting his hump—going above and beyond for his health (i.e. when his weight kept creeping up, it wasn't his fault). Now fast forward to Week Seven in The WOW! ℞: He did the exact same 30-minute elliptical workout as a "cool down" immediately following a vigorous two-hour treadmill-circuit training session! It wasn't until he got in shape that he realized how deep in denial he'd actually been.

The following guidelines will help you in your exercise program:

- Get to bed one hour earlier than your usual bedtime.
- Wake up one hour earlier than usual to get in your morning workout.
- Exercise twice a day at the same times each day, six days a week.
- Aerobic exercise an hour each morning.
- Push-Pull-Twist training or other circuit training an hour every other PM plus aerobic exercise or a recreational sport an hour every other PM.
- Exercise at the upper edge of your envelope. You should truly feel that you are pushing yourself hard and be breathing hard enough that you find it difficult to carry on a conversation.
- Journal the time you spend on exercise in three separate columns: 1. vigorous (aerobic exercise equal to or more intense than jogging); 2. moderate (aerobic exercise less intense than jogging); 3. circuit (anaerobic/aerobic circuit weightlifting).

Total all columns every week to make sure you're on track, getting in 10 to 12 hours of exercise each week.

HOW MUCH EXERCISE IS THERE IN THE WOW! ℞?

There is enough exercise to burn about 1 percent of your weight per week—all fat—and get your heart in peak condition. But remember, dietary restrictions are key as some exercisers compensate by increasing food intake and slightly decreasing their resting metabolism. The

WOW! ℞ caloric intake was formulated to take off an additional 0.5 percent for a grand total of 1.5 percent weight loss per week over the first 10 weeks, before the weight loss slows down a bit.

Okay, let's tackle the math. Not including The WOW! ℞ Nutrition Plan, an obese 150-pound person needs to exercise off 1.5 pounds (1 percent); a 200-pounder, 2 pounds (1 percent); a 250-pounder, 2.5 pounds (1 percent); a 400-pounder, 4 pounds of fat per week (1 percent). To accomplish this, The WOW! ℞ Training Plan includes aerobic activities complemented by strength training. You'll push yourself up to, and a bit beyond, your comfort zone, realizing, of course, that it will take a few weeks to really get going.

Be aware: Early in the program, water shifts may delude you into believing that you're losing more than 1.5 percent. Avoid dehydration by drinking liberal amounts of noncaloric beverages, avoid low-sodium levels by salting your food for the first months, and avoid potassium and mineral losses by consuming your full complement of "core foods," including fruits and vegetables. One caveat: A recurring theme in my examinations of obese folks is "pitting edema"—pounds of extra fluid just under ankle and shin skin—in part a consequence of fat impeding lymph flow—so this type of fluid loss is good.

Bottom Line, How Much Exercise is in The WOW! ℞?

Exercise up to one hour each morning and an hour each evening, six days a week for individuals desiring the ultimate results, the most dramatic fat loss as quickly as is safely possible. Individuals desirous of a more gradual loss of excess fat, or those who do not need to lose as much fat in order to achieve the desired results, can embark on this program with lower amounts of exercise each day.

Throw away your preconceived notions; to the shock and disbelief of every weight-loss "expert"—and almost everybody else—2 to 2.5 hours of exercise a day was tolerated by every single one of the morbidly obese *Biggest Loser* home participants. By the two-month mark, as fat fell off at an average rate of two-thirds of a pound a day, this level of exercise was no longer tolerated—it was savored! But we're getting ahead of ourselves.

What Would It Take to Lose 1 Percent Each Week from Exercise?

Presume you weigh 200 pounds. Divide your current weight (in pounds) by 100 to calculate 1 percent. For example, 1 percent of 200 pounds equals 2 pounds. Fat is about 3,500 calories per pound. So, to lose 2 pounds of fat (at 3,500 calories per pound), you need to burn an extra 7,000 calories from exercise each week. (As luck would have it, the compensatory appetite increase is far less when you exercise off an extra 7,000 calories as compared to eating 7,000 calories less.)

As it turns out, whether you weigh 150, 200, 300, or even 400 pounds, you require the exact same amount of weekly exercise to lose fat amounting to 1 percent of your body's weight. If you're twice as heavy, you burn approximately twice the calories for the same exercise; but remember, if you're twice as heavy, you must also lose twice as much fat to lose 1 percent of your weight.

How Does Exercise Intensity Affect the Amount of Weight You'll Lose?

How many hours of moderate (3 mph) walking does an obese adult have to do in order to lose fat amounting to 1 percent of their body weight each week? It's 33.3 hours per week!

Let's do the math, staying with the example of a 200-pound person (but remembering that the calculation is exactly the same for every other weight): 7,000 calories divided by 210 *additional* calories exercised off per hour (300 calories an hour burned during moderate walking minus 90 calories an hour [your baseline—the number of calories you'd burn if you'd stayed on the couch and watched TV—see Table 7.1]) equals 33.3 hours of walking per week.

Table 7.1 Calories Expended per Hour from Various Activities and Exercises

Weight (lbs)	150	175	200	250	300	350	400
Sleep	60	70	80	100	120	140	160
TV watching	68	79	90	113	135	158	180
Reading, sitting	90	105	120	150	180	210	240
Reading, standing	120	140	160	200	240	280	320
Yoga, stretch	169	197	225	281	338	394	450
Weightlifting—moderate	225	263	300	375	450	525	600
Weightlifting—vigorous	413	482	550	688	825	963	1,100
Nonstop circuit training	544	635	725	906	1,088	1,269	1,450
Walking—moderate (3 mph)*	225	263	300	375	450	525	600
Walking—brisk (4 mph)*	338	394	450	563	675	788	900
Walking—fast (4.5 mph)*	432	503	575	719	863	1,006	1,150
Jogging (5 mph)*	544	635	725	906	1,088	1,269	1,450
Running (6 mph)*	675	788	900	1,125	1,350	1,575	1,800
Running up stairs*	1,023	1,193	1,363	1,704	2,045	2,385	2,726

*In several places I mention "walking" and "jogging" and imply that it equates to moving 3 and 5 mph respectively; actually, this depends on leg length, stride, age, weight, and posture. Shorter, younger individuals may begin to jog at closer to 4 mph or less (the body has an innate calculator that tells you the exact speed at which jogging becomes more fuel efficient than fast walking).

Now do you see why the average two to three hours a week of walking that the *Biggest Loser* applicants did was of no benefit at all for controlling their weight? You would need to exercise at that level for 5.5 hours a day (33.3 hours divided by six days equals 5.5 hours per day) for a 1 percent weight loss! That's practically a full-time job. Good luck losing fat that way!

How many hours of moderate weightlifting does an obese adult have to do in order to lose fat amounting to 1 percent of body weight each week? Again, 33.3 hours!

It's essentially the same calculation for our model 200-pound obese individual: 7,000 calories divided by 210 extra calories exercised off per hour (300 calories an hour during moderate weightlifting minus 90 calories an hour [your baseline—the number of calories you'd burn if you'd stayed on the couch and watched TV]) equals 33.3 hours of typical weightlifting per week. Divide that by six exercise days per week and you realize—assuming you're the typical American barbell user—that you'd have to pump iron a full 5.5 hours a day to lose 1 percent of your weight. Again, good luck losing fat that way!

Okay, I hear your message: You could increase the intensity a bit.

How many hours of brisk (4 mph) walking do you need to do to lose 1 percent of body weight (all fat) each week? Twenty hours!

Again, you've got to burn off 7,000 calories divided by 360 extra calories exercised off per hour (450 calories an hour walking briskly minus 90 calories an hour—what you'd burn if you stayed on the couch and watched TV). That comes out to a little under 20 hours per week or 3.25 hours a day of brisk walking—again, almost impossible, considering the time demands of life for the typical 21st-century, multitasking adult.

What if you notch up the intensity one more rung?

How many hours of very fast walking (4.5 mph) to lose 1 percent of body weight (all fat) each week? It's 15 hours a week (using the same math as above).

Suddenly you can see possibilities. The average American watches more television a week than this! You'd need to fast walk "only" 2.5 hours a day, six days a week to meet the 1 percent weight-loss-as-fat quota—a tall order to be sure, but vaguely plausible.

How about jogging? Eleven hours per week!

Eureka! You're there! Two hours per day, six days a week! When your resting calorie burn is factored in, the net caloric burn of jogging is threefold higher than a 3 mph walk!

One last trick to increase your calorie burn: split the two hours into morning and evening workouts. This results in more calories burned compared with doing two consecutive hours of exercise. Three 40-minute workout sessions a day might be even better, but that's less practical.

"But I Can't Jog!" You Say?

No problem. Most Americans currently can't jog for more than a few seconds. Amazingly, I've seen highly rated obese NFL linemen who've never run farther than up and back the length of a football field. Most of *The Biggest Loser* contestants had not jogged a single stride since childhood, but that changed quickly, and you, too, will be able to jog within a few short months.

Be aware, however, that there are lots of walking exercises with an equivalent calorie burn to jogging. These are perfect for those who have orthopedic injuries that prevent them from jogging or those who simply want to change their exercise routines. Table 7.2 gives you an idea of calories burned during various "jogging-equivalent" walking exercises.

Do I Need Special Fluid Replacements to Compensate for All the Sweating?

In comfortable clothes and temperate weather, one hour of moderate to vigorous exercise will initially result in the loss of about 1 to 3 pounds

Table 7.2 Calories Expended per Hour from
"Jogging-Equivalent" Walking Exercises

Weight (lbs)	150	200	300	400
Jogging (5 mph)	544	725	1,088	1,450
Walking @ 3 mph up 12.5% grade	544	725	1,088	1,450
Walking @ 3.5 mph up 10% grade	544	725	1,088	1,450
Walking @ 3.8 mph up 8% grade	544	725	1,088	1,450
Walking @ 3.5 mph up 5% grade	544	725	1,088	1,450
with weights on each ankle	(2.5 lbs)	(3 lbs)	(5 lbs)	(6 lbs)

of sweat and 500 to 2,000 mg of sodium. The goal is to replace sweat losses (you should check this at least once: starting weight plus fluids ingested minus amount urinated minus end of exercise weight; remember 1 cup equals .5 of a pound) and sodium losses (lightly salt your food).

- Drink one glass of water 30 minutes pre-exercise; assuming acceptable taste, room temperature tap water (20–60 mg sodium/cup) is superior to bottled water (0–20 mg sodium/cup), "smart water" (0 sodium), or mineral water (0 sodium)
- Drink one glass of water immediately pre-exercise
- Drink one glass of water each 10 to 15 minutes (don't miss these drinks; your thirst is a lousy indicator of your fluid status)
- Anabolic (muscle building) shake immediately post-exercise

Can I Increase My Metabolism?

Yes. Lean (fat-free) tissue determines metabolism, so by simply growing additional lean tissue or, alternatively, teaching your lean tissue to burn fat more efficiently, you effectively rev up your metabolism.

Even when you're sound asleep, your lean tissue keeps blazing through calories. Your liver (27 percent of your resting needs), brain (19 percent), skeletal muscles (18 percent), kidneys (10 percent), and heart (7 percent) guzzle through stored energy. Fat cells, on the other hand, virtually sit still, requiring only minimal fuel for fat-cell functions, including spitting out several hormones affecting satiety, sugar metabolism, and inflammation. It would be nice to add more brain and heart, but these organs have little or no growth potential. So, for practical purposes, the only calorie-guzzling body part we can enlarge is skeletal muscle. Each pound of muscle tacked on burns an extra 30 calories per day at rest. But in reality, it's a challenge to gain muscle, and former wisdom claimed muscle growth was impossible in the face of active caloric deprivation. Amazingly, the average home contestant gained at least 9 (women) to 14 (men) pounds of muscle—a grand slam compared to muscle loss on other weight-loss programs and weight-loss surgeries!

But be wary, the flip side can be unforgiving: If you were to go from regular exercise to no exercise, loss of muscle and downshifts in resting metabolism are inevitable. Less obvious but no less foolhardy, virtually all studied low-calorie medical and fad diets with inadequate exercise leech protein from organs and skeletal muscle for fuel, resulting in the net cannibalization of lean tissue. Of your heroic 60-pound weight loss, 20 or more of that could be lean tissue (including bone, muscle, and water). That's literally a hollow—sunken face—victory. Then, as you fight to maintain the weight loss, the struggle, in part, is because now you're burning hundreds of calories less a day at rest than before just to break even (by some estimates, 20 pounds of lost lean tissue adds up to 280 fewer calories burned a day—14 calories per pound of lean lost). You've also shortchanged your ability to burn extra calories through exercise, because the less muscle you have, the fewer calories that muscle can burn when it's working hard. So if you lose weight by dieting without significant exercise, you've sabotaged yourself. You've set yourself up for defeat.

Let's take a closer look at The WOW! ℞ Exercise Plan.

THE WOW! ℞ EXERCISE PLAN

Step One: Jump-Start Your Morning and Burn Fat

Make your morning workout a ritual!

- Start with a good night's sleep.
- Begin at the same time every day.
- Do your dynamic warm-up.
- Keep at the initial month walk-jog pace.
- Increase speed, intensity, and distance as weeks progress.
- Push yourself to the outer edge of your physical envelope.
- Follow the daily grind.

Never Sacrifice Sleep

Go to bed an hour earlier. Never sacrifice sleep—unless your partner propositions you. A full night's rest is essential for weight loss and a high-performance life. You'll know your body clock is working and that you've gotten adequate rest when you wake up just before the alarm goes off and you feel alert and energetic throughout the day. Besides the fat-loss benefits of The WOW! ℞, there are additional benefits once your sleep pattern has adjusted:

- Your "getting-ready-for-work" time will be slashed to a fraction of the usual. I get out of bed at 5 A.M. and shave while doing alternate hamstring stretches at the sink, then I'm out the door for my morning run. When I get back an hour later, my energy is up and I can literally fly through the remainder of the showering and dressing routine. On mornings I don't run, it never ceases to amaze me how long it takes me to get showered and dressed. It turns out that I'm like a lot of my patients, wasting 30 minutes or more on slow-motion getting-ready rituals.
- Once you get the endorphin high—a couple of months into the

program—you will work faster, think clearer, and make superior decisions. The exercise-induced chemical brain boost literally allows you to work more efficiently; you can compress your 16-hour day into 15 hours—thereby getting back one of the exercise hours—and do a better job!

- One of the really great silver linings of getting healthy and losing fat on The WOW! ℞ is more restful sleep. It turns out that obese individuals are lousy sleepers. Obesity-related sleep problems are usually caused by a variety of factors: depression, anxiety, reflux, asthma, snoring, and low-oxygen spells from obstructed breathing (sleep apnea).

Begin at the Same Time Every Day

Wake up at the same time each morning, an hour earlier than usual, roll out of bed, throw on a hat and sweats, and immediately begin the outdoors walk-jog. Warm up with a fast walk or slow jog for three to five minutes. Coax out a little armpit moisture.

A Dynamic Warm-Up

After you work up a fine sweat, you're ready. Now begin the dynamic flexibility and strengthening drills to fully lubricate each foot, leg, and back muscle and joint for maximum function and injury protection. This dynamic warm-up is funny looking, but important in order to decrease the risk of injuries and soreness.

Ankles First

Start by taking 50 steps in every imaginable ankle position.

1. Slow jog 50 steps with toes up (just on your heels).
2. Toes down (tiptoes).
3. Toes pointed 30 degrees in (pigeon-toed).
4. Toes pointed 30 degrees out (Charlie Chaplin).

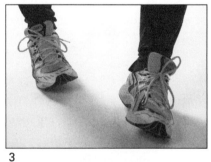

1

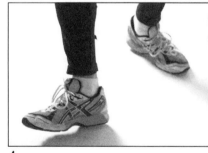

2

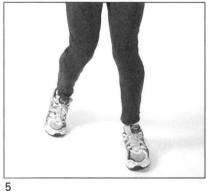

3

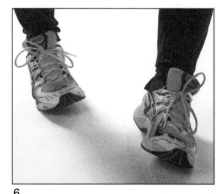

4

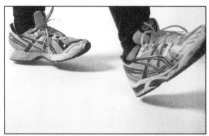

5

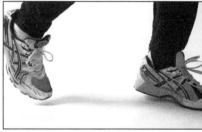

6

5. On the inside of your foot (knock-kneed).
6. And on the outside of your foot (bow-legged).
7. Then, finally, work the Achilles a little more by going 50 paces in a crouched position (keeping back straight).

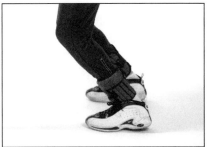

7

Now, the Knees

1. Skip every other step, lifting the thigh parallel to the ground with the foot down.
2. Then straighten out the entire leg—stretch the hamstring—in front of you.

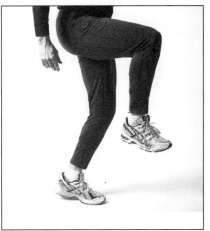

1

These simple "moving" warm-ups, which track athletes do before races, will totally wear you out for the first few months before your conditioning kicks in. Just walk, hands on hips for a few moments. You'll quickly catch your breath and be able to move on to the remaining dynamic stretches.

The important hamstring warm-up is next, aptly termed the "dog-poop-on-shoe" warm-up.

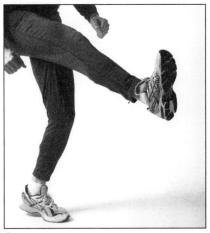

2

3. You maintain a slow jog, each step firmly scraping the sole of the shoe on the ground. It's not so great for maintaining sneaker tread, but it's a key dynamic hamstring and calf waker-upper.

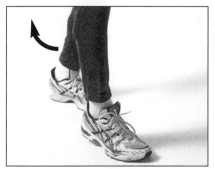

3

4. Next do the butt kick, fully flexing the knee, taking each step with the heel attempting to strike up against your same-side derriere.

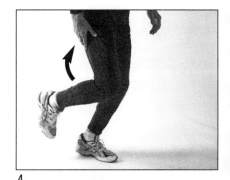

4

Hips/Back

1. At the level of the hip, start with 25 (50 will take some practice) alternating steps with knees so high in air that they actually touch up against your chest.

Once you perform this butt stretch, hip-flexor warm-up, you'll never again criticize those idiotic-looking marching bandleaders.

Next up, 25 hip extensions—they can 1 be a little awkward for nondancers like me—but you'll soon catch on.

2. Hop on the right leg once you've got the left leg as far back in the air behind you as you can, then take a normal step and reverse sides.

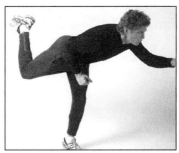

2

3. We're almost done! The back-stretches are last. Sidestep 50 paces with hips facing right, but torso and head twisted forward. Switch sides.

4. Finally, backpedal 10 steps at a reasonable clip, rotating head and torso over the right shoulder to avoid oncoming traffic, parked cars, trees, or potholes. After 10 steps backward, rotate spine so you're looking over the left shoulder. Continue to alternate every 10 paces for a total of 60 paces.

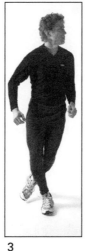
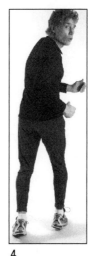

3   4

Congratulations! You've given your running engine a first-rate tune-up. Great things are just over the horizon. Okay, you may look a little crazy to passing motorists. When I was illustrating these funny-looking moves to the home contestants on the UCLA track, we drew our share of incredulous looks from bystanders, but guess what? *The Biggest Losers* caught on quickly, and you'll master this all-purpose flexibility-strengthening program, too. Before long, you'll be able to complete even more strenuous warm-ups with one- and two-legged hops and have lots of energy left for exercise.

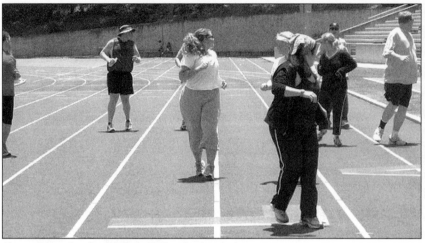

Home team backpedaling (full spinal twist)

The First-Month Morning Walk-Jog Pace

Okay, your joints and muscles are all geared up and oiled, now head toward the most scenic part of your neighborhood, jogging a full block, then fast-walking a few blocks, then jogging again. Within days, your wind will allow you to jog a block alternating with a block of fast walking; progress as you are able. True, you get some cardiovascular benefits from moderate walking (as little as 30 minutes a day), but go back and reread Table 7.1, page 93. Moderate walking doesn't qualify as a "weight-loss" exercise. You need to exercise at the edge of your ability—this is called *intense* exercise. And by the way, the more intense your exercise, the more cardiovascular benefits you receive. You're getting into the intense range during exercise when you're not able to talk comfortably.

Dial down the intensity slightly if at any time you sense the exercise is very hard and you're uncomfortably short of breath. If you become excessively winded, downshift to a slower jog or brisk walk, then, in a minute or two, when you catch your breath, jog at the earlier (tough) pace again. Got the idea? Keep your foot on the accelerator as long as you can to burn extra fuel. Tire, but don't exhaust yourself. Stay on the edge—somewhat hard exertion with regular huffing—but *do not* go over the top—very hard exertion with air gasping. If you experience weird symptoms, such as chest, neck, or jaw pains with exercise, go back and see the doctor who cleared you.

Push Yourself

You've walked/jogged away from home for 30 minutes, now turn around and head back. We're aiming for 4.5 miles or more (survey your routes on your car odometer ahead of time), but make sure the round trip is at least four miles. If not, wake up earlier. If you're going slowly—less than 4 mph—that's okay, but even at the beginner stage, you need to complete a minimum of four miles to call it "one hour" of fat-loss exercise!

The Daily Grind

Back at home, grab your pre-blended anabolic shake (see Section Three for recipes), jump in the shower, and you're off. The morning workout supercharges you; aside from the aforementioned speedy dressed-for-work effect, there's also less need for coffee (one drug and one 15-minute Starbucks stop eliminated), and a newfound focus at work and/or school. At your destination, a static stretch would be ideal, but given the reality of one hour of morning exercise crowding in on your already busy day, a formal warm-down is not absolutely needed. If you do have the inclination, you could do calf and hamstring stretches at stoplights while driving to work or early in your day during phone calls.

Are There Morning Exercise Alternatives?

Scientific studies have measured the amount of calories people burn during various forms of exercise. It turns out that men and women naturally self-select a higher level of exertion—a higher calorie burn—with jogging compared to exercising on equipment such as a stationary bike, elliptical machine, Health Rider, rowing machine, or Nordic Track. Despite burning more calories (and fat) per hour, joggers don't feel that they are exerting themselves more, nor do they feel an ounce more fatigued.

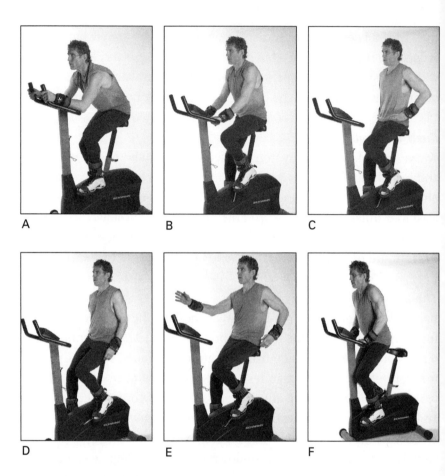

Figure 7.1 At a steady speed and resistance, you burn more calories as you go from fully-supported (A, B) to supported (C, D) to less-supported positions (E, F).

Now you know why I'm so gung ho about the morning walk/jog.

When you have to support all of your body weight (or better yet, increase it by wearing ankle and/or wrist weights) and have to keep yourself balanced, you use more muscles (including your core body muscles for balance) and burn more calories. Is it any wonder, given my goal of maximizing calorie burn per hour, that every exercise you do sitting down or with arms braced on handles is on my "second-tier" list? I recommend these lower calorie-burning exercises be used mainly to break monotony or to gain spiritual points (yoga). However, second-tier exercise does become essential when foot, ankle, or other orthopedic mishaps necessitate nonweight-bearing exercises on a stationary bike or elliptical. When exercising on a stationary bike, recognize that at a steady speed and resistance, you burn more calories as you go from more- to less-supported positions (figure 7.1).

I'm partial to outdoor walk/jogs for various reasons. Jogging outdoors on slightly uneven surfaces into a cool morning breeze burns more calories than a similar treadmill pace. (And no, the return trip with the wind at your back doesn't begin to equal the higher calorie burn incurred while running into the wind.) Getting out of the house eliminates family and work distractions (try to leave your cell phone at home), it's economical (free!), and there's no temptation to lean on the satanic treadmill handrails (they can reduce fat burn by a shocking 20 to 30 percent!).

There are other treadmill negatives, too. Many obese people can't use treadmills because the spinning belt will skip when one's weight crests up over 300 pounds. They're also unsafe while trying to do the moving dynamic flexibility-strengthening warm-ups. And the treadmill isn't as complete an exercise for your body as jogging outdoors; the spinning belt pulls the extended front foot backward with each stride, reducing the hamstring muscle work—that's why competitive runners shun treadmill workouts. Lastly, sprinting and interval speed work on a treadmill are difficult, if not outright unsafe. (I hear you guffawing at the very mention of higher speeds, but just wait and see, in two to three months you are going to be amazed. I don't pretend to understand how this is possible, but I've seen morbidly obese couch potatoes transform into 10K competitors, or even mini-triathlon finishers, in under 12 weeks!)

Striding over fallen leaves while breathing in the crisp morning air versus plodding but going nowhere on a treadmill in a sweaty gymnasium under a wall decorated with television talking heads... is there really any comparison?

Who Should Use a Treadmill?

Even though you can see I'm not a huge fan, there are a number of good reasons why you might want to use a treadmill:

- *Unsafe neighborhoods.* There are some areas of this country that are considered truly unsafe, and some upscale neighborhoods where crimes do occur—everyone certainly remembers the brutal New York City Central Park jogger rape case. Even though that's not a totally acceptable excuse for avoiding outdoor jogging, especially when it's possible to gather like-minded people to run as a group—and lose fat together—there are times when women, especially, and sometimes men, are at risk, particularly when running alone in the dark.
- *Hill work.* Some of us have hills right in our backyards, but many live in perfectly flat locales. True, even the flattest Plains states' towns have streets with moderate grades, but sometimes it's nice to set exact speeds and inclines (plus ankle weights) to achieve the calorie burn of a 5 mph jog at friendly walking speeds.
- *Runner's diarrhea.* I have patients who get diarrhea practically every time they run. Okay, it's hard to argue with the preference for treadmills (near a bathroom!) in that situation.
- *Weather extremes.* It can be tough, and sometimes unsafe, to run in icy, snowy conditions when sidewalks are virtually impassible (I feel your chills; I've spent many winters in Boston, Ann Arbor, Chicago, and Rochester), but remember, exercise in hot and cold environments burns extra calories! The first 15 minutes working out on a near-freezing morning is a bit of a pain, but if you're wearing the right gloves and ski hat, you quickly warm to the task.

Obviously I'm not going to get many endorsement offers to hype indoor gyms or treadmills, but, despite the above, make no mistake, treadmills do allow a good solid workout with a calorie burn in the general ballpark of outdoor jogging. So if, for whatever reason, you don't feel like venturing outdoors, the treadmill is for you.

If You're Not a Morning Person, What Can You Do?

Many of you are night owls, folks whose brains don't function very well until 10 A.M. Owls do their best work in the afternoon and evening. In medicine, we call "owls" *rock 'n' rollers* to differentiate them from the "larks," the stereotypical stockbrokers, lawyers, doctors, and truckers who rise at 5 A.M. or earlier, Saturdays included, annoyingly raring to go. It may be difficult during the first several days to drag your body out of bed early, but just accept it and climb out of bed. Decide that hitting the snooze button on your alarm is not an option. *Force yourself out of bed.*

After a few days, you will be tired earlier in the evening, and your circadian rhythm will start to adjust. Actually, daily morning exercise may be the perfect way to naturally align your circadian rhythm to the 8-to-5 grind. (You also save the cost of that espresso machine and the extra teeth cleanings to get rid of coffee stains.)

Step Two: Ritualistic Afternoon Exercise

Why Work Out in the Afternoon?

Admittedly, exercising two times a day takes real dedication. Frankly, two years ago I'd have scoffed at the suggestion that any of us hourly working stiffs—that includes stay-at-home moms—could possibly squeeze in a second hour of exercise each day. That was before the 36 home-only participants, before I witnessed working moms average two hours of exercise a day—even when they knew there was no chance they'd win prize money—before I watched in awe as real people (a procurement coordinator, a doctor, a hair stylist, a construction worker, a reading consultant, a police officer, a minister, a nurse, a teacher, a waitress, a student, a coroner, a pharmaceutical rep, among others) consistently made the time and changed their lives.

- Make your afternoon workout a ritual as well: Do Push-Pull-Twist training (detailed in Chapter Nine) three afternoons/evenings a week to maximize calorie burning and balance/agility while adding calorie-guzzling and body-toning muscle.

- Do fun, competitive, camaraderie-filled social sports or aerobic activities three afternoons/evenings a week to seamlessly assist the development of active lifetime skills that are a vital part of weight maintenance.
- All things being equal, upright activities, such as speed walking, running, skiing, skating, and stair climbing utilize more energy than "nongravity" sports, such as biking, swimming, rowing, or "bench-sitting" weightlifting.

Enhanced Daily Living

On a practical basis, when it comes to burning off large quantities of fat, aerobic exercise is the main mover. After the body gets in endurance shape, it's possible to increase the metabolic rate tenfold to twentyfold! Translation: This means going from a calorie burn of 100 while watching TV to a 1,000-plus hourly burn with peak exercise. Ultra-endurance athletes burn over 10,000 calories a day. Many previously sedentary, morbidly obese *Biggest Loser* contestants exercised off over 3,500 calories (1 pound of fat) a day within a week of starting rigorous exercise. Endurance training, like resistance training—even with no net-muscle growth— also bumps up metabolism, presumed secondary to aerobically challenged-muscle-producing-specialized energy-devouring enzymes.

In terms of positive health spin-offs, the sky's the limit with aerobic exercise. Mood and intelligence augmentation; heart disease, diabetes, Alzheimer's, and cancer prevention; and treatment of a host of disabling conditions, such as arthritis and chronic pain.

Chapter Eight

Push-Pull-Twist (PPT) Training: The Last Piece of the Fat-Loss Puzzle

Anyone can purchase a pair of running shoes and hit the local park for a free aerobic workout. No such luck for strength training. You have to either ante up for a gym membership, a trainer to walk you through the byzantine exercise machines, or a strength-training self-help book—almost all of which recommend gym equipment that could set you back thousands of dollars. Even if you're lucky enough to have a little extra space in your garage or an entire spare room, why bother cluttering it with a "universal" or other advertised-on-TV machine that has a new and improved capacity to bench-press 400 pounds when you can barely do one lousy push-up?

Do you really want to pay two grand to exercise on indoor machines that encourage sitting and one-dimensional lifting and make it impossible to do integrated whole-body balance work? I don't think so. There's a better, more economical way—a way of exercising on your feet in three dimensions, your entire body balanced and working in concert to accomplish resistance movements.

This amazing home gym fits in your house or apartment and is as effective as the most elaborate built-in weight rooms of the rich and famous. Best of all, every one of you can afford it!

THE PUSH-PULL-TWIST HOME GYM

How Much Space Do You Need?

- 8 × 8 feet of open floor space while using the equipment
- A portion of one closet to store the equipment

How Much Will It Cost?

For $350 you can buy all the gear you'll need to have a home gym guaranteed to rival that of any tycoon (Plymouth Rock hen not included).

What Items Do You Need?

- Rubberized nonroll hexagonal dumbbells—3-, 5-, 10-, 15-, 20-pound matched pairs ($150)
- Swiss ball ($20 for economical varieties, $35 for thicker-skinned brands). Select the size that allows you to sit on top of a 90 percent inflated ball with your feet comfortably on the ground and your thighs parallel to the floor. Buy a larger ball if you have long legs for your height, chronic back problems, or are planning to use the Swiss ball as an office chair. The following are the recommended sizes by height:

  45cm (18-inch) ball for those less than 5' 0" tall
  55cm (22-inch) ball for those who are 5' 0" to 5' 5"
  65cm (26-inch) ball for those 5' 5" to 6' 0"
  75cm (30-inch) ball for anyone 6' 0" and over

- Thick rubber instability mat—measuring 16″ by 20″ ($50)
- Jump rope ($15)
- Doorjamb pull-up bar—*must be screwed in,* not compression attached, for obvious safety reasons ($20)
- Rubber resistance bands ($30 for two—thicker, higher resistance bands cost a bit more)
- Adjustable, strap-on ankle (10-pound) and wrist (5-pound) weights (weight is adjustable in half-pound increments by adding or subtracting lead bars) ($50)

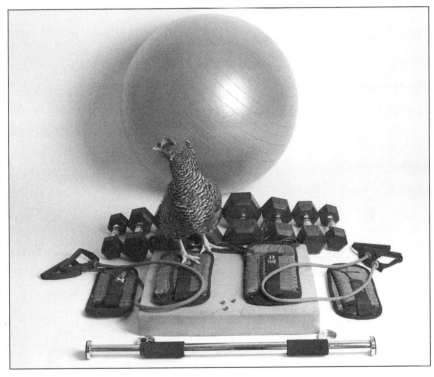

The PPT home gym.

Stick to the Game Plan: Lose Fat—Not Muscle, Water, or Bone

Can you imagine how crazy it would be to drop weight by sacrificing vital body structures? Shockingly, that's exactly what the vast majority of people on very low-calorie diets or weight-loss pills do. Very low-calorie fad diets can literally cannibalize chunks of muscle; they have no muscle transformational value, and thus do not rev up metabolism. In patients receiving the two most common gastric bypass surgeries, fully 25 to 50 percent of their weight loss is lean tissue! When you eliminate metabolically active tissue, you sabotage any chance for lasting fat loss and health gains. Plus, studies show that even a modest 10 percent weight loss via diet alone can result in significant, 2 percent-plus spine and hip-bone loss—common body locations for later-in-life osteoporotic fractures.

If you want to retain, and often even gain, muscle and spinal- and hip-bone mass during weight loss, optimize body shape and tone—even facial wrinkles are due, in part, to loss of facial bone and muscle—and maintain fat loss, then you need to work both strength (white meat) and endurance (red meat) muscle fibers. Even trim runners in great cardiovascular shape (their red-meat muscle is in tiptop condition) need to lift weights or risk inexorable age-related weakening and shrinkage of the body-shaping white meat.

Outdoor aerobics address the red-meat endurance muscle; PPT training addresses the white (fast-twitch) muscle that packs a force five times higher than the dark (endurance) muscle, but fatigues much more quickly. In case you're curious, endurance muscle is dark because of its nonstop energy-generating, iron-rich mitochondria; white (power) muscle contains 10 seconds worth of instantly available energy—one all-out sprint—but few red-tinted, nonstop energy-generating mitochondria.

Different people respond quite differently to weightlifting because of individual hormonal, genetic, age, nutritional, and training profiles. And that's fortunate, because very few women (and not many men) desire Schwarzenegger bulk. Besides, ladies, it cannot happen even if you lift very heavy weights—unless you inject testosterone. PPT training will on average increase your muscle mass, but more importantly, rest assured, it will totally transform the muscle! It will get stronger, firmer, and more efficient at burning fat.

We'll ease into PPT training, as opposed to the outdoor aerobics, where I asked you to go all out starting on day one. The first month we'll emphasize form without any heavy lifting. The second month we'll add extra balance and twist components. Then, in month three, we'll jack up the resistance and really get a legitimate pump going. The bottom line? In order to retain or gain muscle mass (critical for a strong, balanced, flexible body and a revved-up metabolism) and muscle shape (critical for cosmetics), you can't afford to ignore this explosive white muscle. Novices should avoid adding excessive weight or doing exhaustive weightlifting during the first months of The WOW! ℞. Some soreness is okay; painful stiffness is a sign of excessive muscle damage.

The Science Behind PPT Training

Calories Burned
Standard weightlifting—lifting the heaviest weight you can manage with good form six to 12 times, with minutes of rest before repeating the whole process another two or more times—and eating an excess of calories with adequate protein is the best way to build muscle. Of course this approach isn't right for dieters. Standard weightlifting isn't a big calorie burner (there's too much rest/recovery time) and, again, to maximize muscle hypertrophy (strength), you need a *surplus* of calories.

PPT training strikes a compromise. Compared to standard weightlifting, the nonstop PPT exercises burn many more calories per hour (almost equivalent to jogging) and, therefore, are more conducive to fat loss. It must be recognized, however, that because of the caloric restriction and the drastically reduced rest/recovery time of PPT exercises, muscle growth is not guaranteed. Still, four-fifths of contestants had muscle growth under these circumstances. One participant, dejected because he couldn't lose as much weight as the other males—he'd lost "only" 47 pounds—had really lost 61 pounds of fat; his "weight" loss was a lot less because he had *gained* 14 pounds of lean tissue! (A more in-depth evaluation revealed he'd lost 76 pounds of normally hydrated fat tissue—fat clings onto water totaling about 20 percent of its weight—and gained about 27 pounds of muscle!) That's an enormous advantage over other weight-loss approaches, where up to 25 to 50 percent of the weight lost is lean tissue—not fat!

Biochemistry

PPT training "works out" the anaerobic energy systems simultaneously with the endurance systems, inducing a unique array of enzymatic changes. These cell signals are responsible for maintaining muscle mass, optimizing the disposal of sugar, fat, harmful cholesterol, and inflammation signals while milking brain cells for "feel-good" neurotransmitters. Given the potent mood-elevating and appetite-suppressing properties of exercise—not to mention the emotional boost of throwing out all of your "fat" clothes—in my experience, a gratifying percentage of depressed patients (but certainly not all) who adopt a regular exercise routine no longer require pharmaceutical mood-enhancement drugs (some of which tend to increase appetite).

Increased Baseline Metabolism

Remember how bears cuddle up in a cave or curl up in a hollowed-out tree and drop off to sleep for months at a time? They must downshift their metabolism, markedly lowering their body temperature and heartbeat, to obviate excessive fat loss. Bears still lose up to 40 percent of body weight during these prolonged winter slumbers, but without their metabolic adjustments they'd lose far more. PPT training with adequate protein in the diet helps negate the human "hibernation" phenomenon—the much-ballyhooed, but still controversial, plateau phase when weight loss is less than expected based on calculated dietary intake versus one's exercise and activity caloric expenditures. This beneficial effect may be mediated by:

- **Enzymatic Enhancements.** When you start PPT training, you flick an invisible switch that causes the cellular engines of white-meat muscle to rev higher than its "couch potato" counterpart. Translation: Even if you don't gain a speck of muscle, strength training bumps up metabolism, presumably by inducing specialized energy-guzzling enzymes.

- **Muscle Retention.** Calorie-restricted diets or weight loss by means of weight-loss pills are a veritable metabolic torpedo, sending muscles the same "melt-away" chemical message as cancer and HIV. Strength and aerobic training may block this "sick" signal.

- **Muscle Enlargement.** A pound of enzymatically jived muscle gained may translate into an extra 30 calories burned per day, and that, in turn, translates into over 10,000 extra calories, or 3 pounds of extra fat, disposed of each year. As previously mentioned, the majority gained muscle during weight loss and some participants gained weight in the MAINTAIN! phase, with tests confirming their extra pounds were muscle tissue—another concrete example exposing weight as a misleading indicator of health. Lose fat, not weight. How many times can I repeat that?

Injury Pre-hab

You must log a lot of exercise hours to lose fat and subsequently keep it off. Strength training helps prevent injuries. Although we tend to give weightlifting credit only for muscle enhancement, it also fortifies bones, ligaments (which hook up bone to bone), tendons (which hook up muscle to bone), as well as connective tissue inside muscle. A prime example: While a 2 percent decrease in lumbar spine density is routinely reported when losing only 5 to 10 percent of weight via diet, the at-home participants either maintained (women) or *gained* lumbar bone density (men, 5 percent). This was a shocker! Bone gain during weight loss has never before been reported. And to have it happen while losing a dramatic amount of weight—essentially all fat—was a scientific head turner.

Symmetrical Strengthening

Lopsided strength is not good; the body functions best when muscles are symmetrically strong and balanced. I had an ex-pro ballplayer who came into my office complaining of back pain. He routinely knocked out a "jillion" sit-ups daily (predominantly a stomach-muscle endurance exercise) without doing a single "strength" sit-up or performing even a few reverse sit-ups or other back-strengthening exercises. He had a pathologic muscle imbalance. Or how about the "spinning" faithful (cycling is predominantly a "push" quad endurance exercise) who never intersperse any hamstring "pull" endurance exercises or any quad or ham-strength training? Or the office worker who hunches over a computer eight hours a day without ever working the opposing high back muscles? And, of course, we all know weightlifters that are fixated on the "mirror" muscles—the biceps, the pectorals, and the abs—and have weak backs supported by chicken legs.

Enhanced Daily Living

PPT training has myriad positive spin-offs, from less anxiety and depression to enhanced sexual prowess. When obvious strength and balance benefits appear, it's often self-perpetuating. A whole new world of activities opens up.

Push-Pull-Twist (PPT) Training—Beginner's Guide

- Have a home gym. (Even if you prefer exercising in a commercial gym for camaraderie, you now have a fallback option when you're rushed for time.)
- Train with a partner(s), if possible.
- Do aerobics of some sort, preferably an outdoor walk-jog, for 30

minutes as a warm-up.

- Focus on the opposing muscles of eight major body motions—16 exercises total (this is the antidote to lopsided strength).
- Do "push" exercises immediately followed by "pull" exercises, then alternate upper-body with lower-body exercises to allow the muscles involved time to recharge without ever having to stop exercising! (Table 8.1).
- Start from the top of the body and move down.
- Press the weight up against gravity quickly, but let it down very very slowly. If you rush the exercise—as most exercisers do by quickly dropping the weight with the pull of gravity—the exercise becomes easier to complete, but you'll need more weight to challenge yourself, which increases joint stress and injury risk.
- Do three-dimensional total-body free-weight exercises, not one- or two-dimensional limited-body-involvement (sitting) machine exercises.
- Never stop moving!

The Learning Curve

Obese strength-training novices need to follow this routine:

First Month

- Work eight major joint movements using a total-body approach.
- Do 12 repetitions of each exercise.
- Use only moderate weight (see pages 123 and 124 for guidance).
- Take one second to smoothly power through the hard part (concentric contraction) of the lift—where the barbell or your body weight is being lifted—and three or four seconds to slowly lower the weight during the easy part (eccentric contraction), where gravity helps move the weight.
- Make the slow, controlled descent as smooth as possible; movements

should be fluid, never jerky.
- Don't hold your breath during exercise. Attempt to breathe out (exhale) during the hard portion of the exercise and breathe in (inhale) during the easy part. Don't panic if you occasionally get this backward – breathing regularly is the overriding objective here!
- Contract muscles quickly (explosively) on ascent (against gravity).
- Move from one exercise to the next quickly (in under 10 seconds).
- These exercises should take less than 25 minutes to perform.
- Stay adequately hydrated.
- Consume properly timed post-workout nutrition with proper macronutrients—an anabolic shake or meal (see Chapter Seven and Section Three for details on food timing, nutrition, and recipes).

This hybrid strength-endurance circuit training maximizes the number of calories expended. Remember, traditional muscle-building regimens have you actually lifting weights for only seven or eight minutes per hour, resulting in an hourly calorie burn that's less than half of a five-miles-per-hour jog.

Everybody seems confused about whether to lift weights first, then do aerobics, or vice versa. The bottom line for dieters: Do the hardest, most rigorous, highest-calorie-burning-per-minute exercise first. At this stage, it's the aerobics. Similar confusion exists regarding what percent of your workout should be aerobics versus weightlifting. Again, for that excess fat, three-quarters or more of the exercise time needs to be the hardest, highest-calorie-burning-per-minute endeavor—the walk-run exercise at this stage. Later, as fat melts off, your goals may shift, and toning and outright muscle hypertrophy (strength) may now top your wish list. You'd therefore adjust your caloric intake upward and retool your exercise approach, alternating endurance, interval, and weight training.

Second Month

Where applicable, we'll make the exercises more difficult by adding twist or balance components; the more muscle groups involved, the tougher the workout, the greater the calorie burn, and the greater your coordination benefit.

Third and Fourth Months

- Increase to two sets of 12 repetitions of each exercise.
- Use progressively more challenging resistance. (*Challenging* means a weight you wouldn't be able to do many more than 12 repetitions if you tried.)
- Keep added weight light enough so that you can complete at least 8 to 12 repetitions with perfect form.
- These exercises should take less than 45 minutes to perform.
- Turn up the heat: Progressively add more resistance until the muscle is overworked (*progressive overload* is the sports-med term). I can't emphasize this enough: Showing up periodically and cruising through the same old strength-training routine with the same amount of weights does not get the job done.

Fifth Month

You're almost an expert now!

- Increase to three sets of each exercise—if you wish (optional).
- Continue to progressively add weight when the routine becomes too easy.
- Combine single-joint moves into unique advanced multi-joint exercises.
- Get your family and friends involved.

PUSH-PULL-TWIST TRAINING—STEP-BY-STEP GUIDE

Beginner's Plan: Month One

On Monday, Wednesday, and Friday in the late afternoon or evening, after you complete a half hour of aerobics, do the 16 exercises shown in Tables 8.1 and 8.2. One set (12 repetitions) with only modest resistance and perfect form, allowing only 10 seconds between exercises. This first month of beginner's PPT training should take a little over 20 minutes.

Master the exercises during the first few weeks with only a modest amount of added resistance. Increased resistance, explosive movements, balance maneuvers, and twists will be added in subsequent months.

Safety first! Heavy weightlifting early in an aggressive weight-loss program for sedentary obese adults is counterproductive, with unnecessary risks for injuries. After you master proper form and wake up your power muscles, routine strength training will become a vital component of fat-loss maintenance and injury prevention.

Begin Starter Weights

During the first month, as you embark on your Push-Pull-Twist strength training and master perfect form, lower weight immediately if the suggested weights in Table 8.1 or 8.2 are too difficult, and add weight if you can do 12 repetitions with absolutely no sweat (and you feel you could do another 5 reps).

Table 8.1 Female Beginner Starter Weights

Push-Pull Exercises	RESISTANCE		
	Ankle Weights (lbs)	Wrist Weights (lbs)	Barbells/ Tube (lbs)
Top Shoulder			
#1—Military press	3	2–5	5 lb set
#2—Chin-up	3	2–5	
Waist			
#3—Reverse sit-up	3	2–5	5 lb set
#4—Sit-up[a]	3	2–5	
Front Shoulder			
#5—Swiss ball bench	3	2–5	5 lb set
#6—Reverse ball bench	3	2–5	
Hip/Buttock			
#7—Donkey kick[a]	3	2–5	
#8—Knee up	3	2–5	
Side Shoulder			
#9—Angel wing	3	2–5	
#10—Reverse angel wing	3	2–5	1 tube[b]
Knee			
#11—Mat squat	3	2–5	
#12—Butt kick	3	2–5	
Elbow			
#13—Tricep press	3	2–5	3 lb set
#14—Curl	3	2–5	3 lb set
Ankle			
#15—Heels up	3	2–5	10 lb set
#16—Toes up	3	2–5	10 lb weight[c]

[a] Initially, this may be difficult to do for 12 repetitions, even with no added weight.
[b] Start with the lowest-resistance tubing.
[c] Place this weight on a thick rubber mat as illustrated in photos.

Table 8.2 Male Beginner Starter Weights

	RESISTANCE		
Push-Pull Exercises	Ankle Weights (lbs)	Wrist Weights (lbs)	Barbells/ Tube (lbs)
Top Shoulder			
#1—Military press	5	5	10 lb set
#2—Chin-up	5	5	
Waist			
#3—Reverse sit-ups	5	5	10 lb set
#4—Sit-ups[a]	5	5	
Front Shoulder			
#5—Swiss ball bench	5	5	10 lb set
#6—Reverse ball bench	5	5	5 lb set
Hip			
#7—Donkey kick[a]	5	5	
#8—Knee up	5	5	
Side Shoulder			
#9—Angel wing	5	5	
#10—Reverse angel wing	5	5	2 tubes[b]
Knee			
#11—Mat squat	5	5	10 lb set
#12—Butt kick	5	5	
Elbow			
#13—Tricep press	5	5	5 lb set
#14—Curl	5	5	10 lb set
Ankle			
#15—Heels up	5	5	15 lb set
#16—Toes up	5	5	20 lb weight[c]

[a] Initially, this may be difficult to do for 12 repetitions, even with no added weight.
[b] Start with the lowest-resistance tubing.
[c] Place this weight on a thick rubber mat as illustrated in photos.

PPT TRAINING—STEP-BY-STEP—MONTH ONE

Top Shoulder Push-Pulls: Exercises 1 and 2

Top shoulder push-pulls are vital for protecting the rotator cuff, one of the most common—and debilitating—injuries caused by everyday over-use or accidents, such as lifting something from the back seat of your car, falling down, or walking your dog and getting yanked by the leash when an unexpected animal encounter occurs.

Exercise 1: Top Shoulder Push (Military Press)

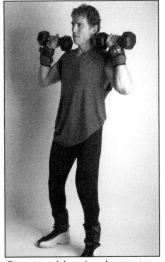

1. Start position: Stand, holding dumb-bells at shoulder height, just to the outside of each shoulder, palms fac-ing forward with elbows fully flexed below your wrists. Keep knees slightly bent.
2. Push dumbbells directly upward until your arms are fully extended over-head, hold for one count (a "count" is approximately one second).
3. Slowly lower (count two).
4. Continue to slowly lower (counts three and four).
5. The instant you return to start posi-tion (at "end" of count four), push dumbbells up again. Slowly count out 2–2-3-4, 3–2-3-4, 4–2-3-4, etc., as you repeat 12 times.

Start position (and count four)

One set (12 reps, about 4 seconds per repetition) takes about 60 sec-onds to complete. The natural four-beat rhythm that exercisers choose is often faster than 1 second per beat, so strive to slow down the easier

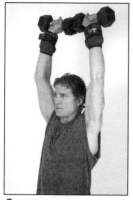

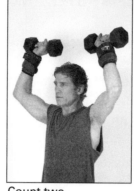

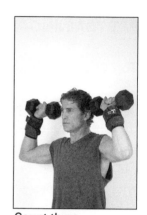

Count one	Count two	Count three

gravity-assisted part of the exercise to at least 3 seconds. This makes all the exercises you'll do much more difficult. And when the difficulty of any lift is increased by slowing down the easy phase—rather than increasing the weight—muscle and joint injuries are decreased.

Exercise 2: Top Shoulder Pull (Chin-Up)

This is a version of the old high school pull-up, with an assist from the floor (you can also choose to rest your feet on a low stool or chair in front of you).

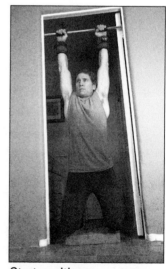

Start position

1. Start position (make sure the door-jamb pull-up bar is screwed in securely at a level that allows you to hang down): Holding onto the bar with a wide overhand grip, hang with your knees an inch or so above the rubber mat, as shown. Place your tiptoes toward the back of the mat, your knees bent and legs limp.

2. Pull up! Get your chin up to the bar (count one) (hopefully you live in a more modern house than I do, with

126

higher doorjams). If you get stuck, use your legs to give yourself enough of a boost to get your chin up to the bar. Keep working. These are tough. Sadly, only a tiny fraction of Americans can do even one real pull-up. You will soon join that elite fraternity.

3., 4. Very slowly lower your body (counts two and three).

5. Return to start position (count four), arms and shoulders fully extended, hanging from the bar, with legs again limp underneath. Knees are still a few

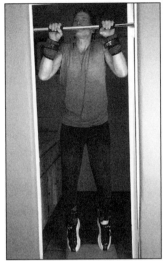

Count one

inches off of the mat. Pull up again. Count out as you repeat 12 reps. Initially, you'll need to keep your toes firmly on the ground and "cheat" a bit with your legs.

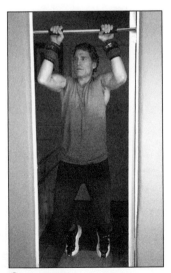

Count two

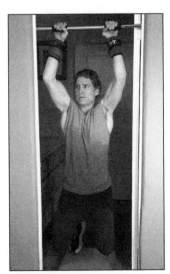

Count three

Waist Push-Pulls: Exercises 3 and 4

The torso pull (sit-up) is the mother of all core conditioning. Despite being perhaps the best-known exercise, many well-intentioned exercisers are confused about whether to focus on endurance (lots of sit-ups) or strength (sets of 12 repetitions of progressively more difficult sit-ups). Conversely, the reverse sit-up may be the least known and most under-utilized pre-hab core exercise.

Exercise 3: Waist Push (Reverse Sit-Up)

1. Start position: Stand with feet shoulder-width apart, knees locked straight, holding light barbells in your hands by your sides.
2. Keeping knees straight, bend forward at the hips, allowing barbells to slowly lower toward the top of your feet (count one). Pull your shoulders back to maintain proper position, especially if you tend to hunch. Add resistance at a snail's pace, allowing time for the lower back to strengthen. Keep arms and knees straight.

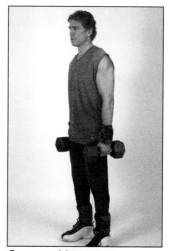

Start position

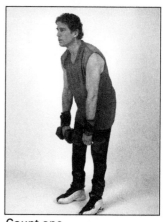

Count one

3. Continue slow descent with gravity (count of two).

4. Do not pause or bounce at bottom of the exercise, when barbells are held over the tops of the shoelaces (count three). Never exceed beyond a mild stretch throughout the back thigh/hamstrings/low back. This means "tight" individuals may not get barbells much past the mid-shins or knees in some cases. If you are one of these "half-jointed" folks don't despair. Your double-jointed yoga teacher is not healthier than you are, based on how many fingers he or she can place on the floor in a straight-leg toe touch. But you can improve your muscle function, and possibly pre-hab injuries, by being as stretched as you can get.

5. Straighten up with picture-perfect posture and extend just slightly backward (count four). Count out as you repeat 12 times. Discontinue if you experience low-back pain.

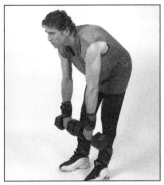

Count two

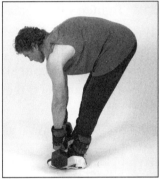

Count three

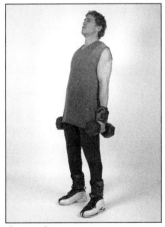

Count four

Exercise 4: Waist Pull (Sit-Up)

1. Start position: Lie flat on your back, rear end at bottom of mat, feet flat on floor, knees bent at 90 degrees, hands down at your sides. (I know the chicken gag is a little tired now, suffice it to say she puts out an egg a day but demands quality time in return...)

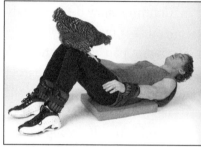

Start position

2. Tighten your stomach muscles and, keeping your upper back straight, inhale and pull torso up to a 60-degree angle off the floor (if your fingers were cupped around your ears, your elbows would touch your knees) (count one). If you don't have ankle weights on, you'll need to stick your toes under a pair of dumbbells or a couch to keep your soles firmly on the floor. Avoid jerky motion.

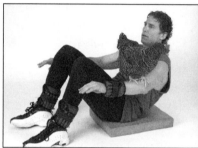

Count one

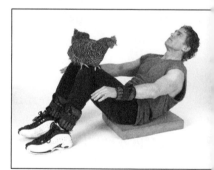

Count two

3. Hold this 60-degree position for a split second, then exhale as you slowly descend (count of two).

4. Continue slow descent (count three)—speedy "momentum" sit-ups increase back strain and rely more on thigh muscles.

5. Descend until your torso is parallel to the floor and the lower back just barely makes contact with the mat (count four), but don't rest your shoulders down on the ground; keep your abs tense and begin the next sit-up. Count out as you repeat 12 times.

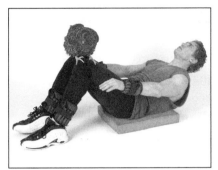

Count three

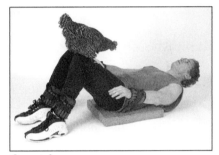

Count four

Don't panic if you can't do 12 reps. Just keep perfect form and persevere until your abdominal muscles wake up. Stop if you feel back pain! Most obese individuals have weak abs and are mechanically disadvantaged—upper body fat makes sit-ups difficult because it's like strapping a barbell to the chest. Meanwhile, waist fat may structurally prevent even a fit obese person from doing a legitimate sit-up.

Keeping your hands down by your sides makes the sit-up easier. Cross your arms across the chest, or cup your fingers around the ears for progressively more challenging sit-ups. Crunches—partial sit-ups moving from a 15- to a 30-degree elevation—are easier and

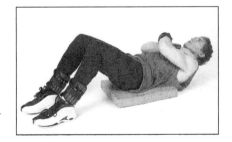

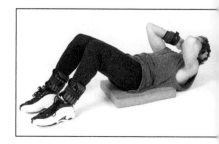

burn fewer calories than an equally paced 60-degree sit-up. Those annoying guys who brag that they do 200 sit-ups every morning? They're usually doing the partial crunches using their hip flexor muscles, typically with rapid up-back-herky-jerky form. And although they develop muscle endurance, their ab muscles may be surprisingly weak.

Front Shoulder Push-Pulls: Exercises 5 and 6

Front shoulder pushes are critical for self-protection (i.e., to simply catch yourself if you fall forward) and, cosmetically, they determine chest size and firmness. Shoulder pulls are a godsend for anyone who is paid to hunch over a tyrannical computer screen all day long or for anyone who tends to slouch.

Exercise 5: Front Shoulder Push (Swiss Ball Bench)
This is a dumbbell bench press on a Swiss ball.

1. Start position: Grab a dumb-bell in each hand. Sit atop a Swiss ball, and slowly walk your feet forward to roll yourself down into a lying position on the ball, on your mid-back, with feet flat on the ground for support. Your low back will follow the Swiss ball contour. Hold the dumbbells to the sides of your

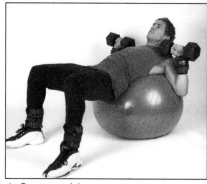

1. Start position

breasts, with elbows under dumbbells (photo 1). If able, now roll even further down and have just your shoulders in contact with the Swiss ball, a harder position because you must tense up all the abdominal muscles and form an abdominal "plank" (photo 3).

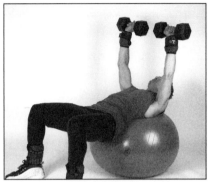

2. Count one (easier)

Obviously, you'll initially use a ridiculously low dumbbell weight while getting the hang of getting on and off of a Swiss ball while holding dumbbells.

2. Push arms directly upward until they are fully extended (count one).

3. Lower weight back down slowly (count two).

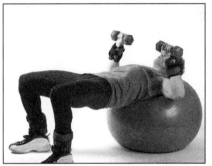

3. Start position (harder)

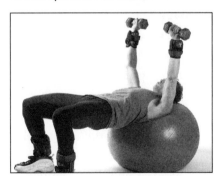

4. Count one (harder)

4. Continue slow descent (count three).

5. Continue slow descent (count four) until you return to start position and immediately repeat the lift. Count out as you repeat 12 times.

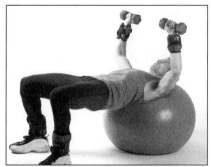

Count two (harder)

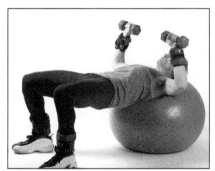

Count three (harder)

Exercise 6: Front Shoulder Pull (Reverse Bell Bench)

1. Start position: Lay face down, lower chest on top of a Swiss ball, legs spread. Initially, it's okay to slide your feet flush against the base of a wall for stability. Ideally, the Swiss ball is sized to allow your arms to hang straight down without touching the floor. The Swiss ball in the photo is a little too small; my arms should be able to hang down all the way, elbows straightened, without hitting the

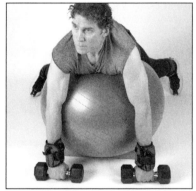

Start position

floor, so I've inserted the rubber mat beneath for a little extra height. Grip dumbbells lying on the floor, palms pointing toward your feet.

2. Now lift your arms—bend the elbows and pull the weights upward on both sides of your body to their respective lateral breast (count one). Concentrate on squeezing the shoulder blades together.

3., 4. Slowly return the weights toward the floor (counts two and three) until arms are extended down back to the start position (end of count four). Count out as you repeat 12 times.

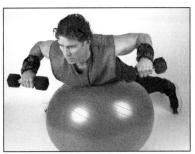

Count one

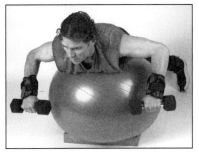

Count two

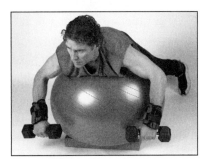

Count three

Hip/Buttock Push-Pulls: Exercises 7 and 8

Hip/buttock push-pulls benefit key muscles in the deservedly much hyped "core," from which all of our arm and leg strength emanates. Although rear-end pushes (the late-night TV "bun" or "glut" exercises) have always been in vogue, the opposite mover, hip/buttock pulls, are uniformly ignored (except for a spillover effect from suboptimal sit-ups).

Exercise 7: Hip/Buttock Push (Donkey Kick)

This is a five-count exercise that needs to be done on the right side alternating with the left side.

1. Start position: Kneel down on the rubber mat on all fours, hands on the front corners of the mat, knees on the back corners.

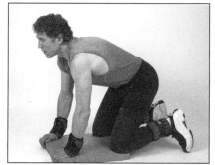

Start position

2. Keeping your knee bent at a 90-degree angle, lift your left thigh up backward until the front part of the thigh is parallel to the floor and hold for a beat (count one).

3. Now push your left foot up toward the ceiling—the thigh should be a pinch past parallel—hold for a beat (count two).

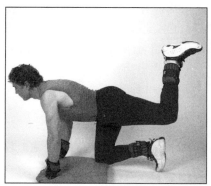

Count one

4., 5. Slowly lower your left leg, while still keeping your knee bent at a 90-degree angle, over the next three seconds (counts three and four) to return to the start position (count five).

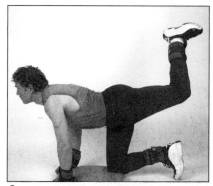

Count two

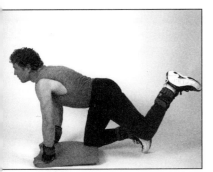

Count three

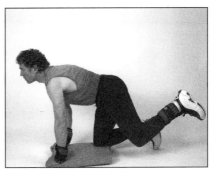

Count four

Repeat using your right leg. Continue to alternate between left and right legs as you count out 12 reps with each leg.

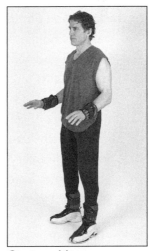

Count five

Exercise 8: Hip/Buttock Pull (Knee Up)

1. Start position: Stand comfortably, feet shoulder-width apart, arms bent at 90 degrees, near a wall or chair for safety, but don't grab hold except for the moment your balance feels iffy!
2. Now lift your left leg up directly to your left breast (not unlike the move you see the leader of a college marching band perform; count one).
3. Slowly lower leg (count two).
4. Continue the slow descent (count three).
5. Return foot to floor (count four).

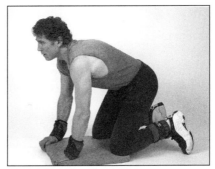

Start position

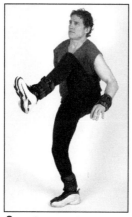
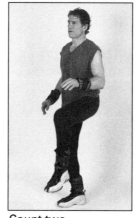
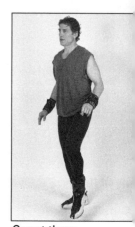

| Count one | Count two | Count three |

Repeat steps 1 through 4 using your right leg. Continue to alternate between left and right legs as you count out 12 reps with each leg.

Side Shoulder Push-Pulls: Exercises 9 and 10

These muscles form an important part of the rotator cuff, and we use them constantly to lift items (from babies to grocery bags) in our daily lives.

Exercise 9: Side Shoulder Push (Angel Wing)

1. Start position: Stand with "soft knees" (knees slightly bent), your 5-pounder wrist weights plus additional light barbells (or cans of soup) if needed hanging by the sides of your thighs with your elbows slightly bent.
2. Raise the upper arms sideways, keeping your elbows fixed in a slightly bent position, until the upper arm is roughly parallel to the floor, the elbows and wrists aligned at shoulder height; pause for a fraction of a second (count one).

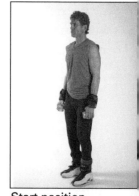

Start position

138

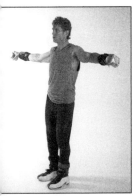
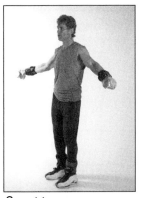
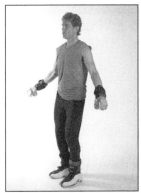

| Count one | Count two | Count three |

3. Slowly lower (count two).
4. Continue to slowly lower (count three).
5. Return to starting position (count four). Count out as you repeat 12 times.

Exercise 10: Side Shoulder Pull (Reverse Angel Wing)

1. Start position: Stand with soft (slightly bent) knees, hold the ends of rubber resistance cord(s) that are firmly double-wrapped around your pull-up bar (securely screwed into doorjamb) with your upper arms raised sideways, elbows slightly bent, elbows and wrists aligned at shoulder height.

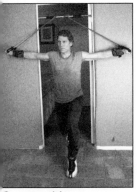
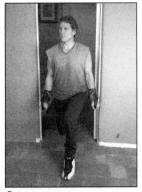
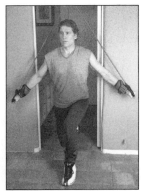

| Start position | Count one | Count two |

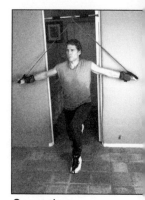

2. Pull down on resistance cord(s), lowering your arms sideways until your hands just touch your thighs. Hold for one beat (count one). (I used two cords in the photo; the more cords or the thicker the cord(s), the more resistance.)

3., 4. Slowly raise your arms back to ward the starting position (counts two and three) until you return to the starting position (count four). Count out as you repeat 12 times.

Count three

Note: Be careful while using bands. Although they are very versatile (you can actually do most of the 16 PPT exercises with bands while away from home or where no weights or gym equipment are available), they can occasionally cause injuries. I've seen several cases where the bands weren't properly secured and snapped back in the face of the startled exerciser.

Knee Push-Pulls: Exercises 11 and 12

Knee push-pulls strengthen the front and back of the thigh—the muscles that serve and protect the knee, hip, and low back. Many athletes and exercisers have sculpted the quads (with copious squats and bike work), while ignoring the posterior thigh, leaving the leg woefully imbalanced and at risk for hamstring and back problems.

Exercise 11: Knee Push ("Mat" Squat)

1. Start position: Stand in front of your rubber mat—its 20-inch-long side is propped upright by weights on each side—with feet shoulder-width apart, toes turned out 15 degrees, and arms at your sides; or if you're not holding weights, you may elect to hold your arms out in front of you to assist your balance.

2. Slow descent (count one). Keeping your heels flat on the floor, slowly lower your butt as though you are going to sit down on a chair.

3. Continue slow descent (count two).

4. Hold for a fraction of a second when your butt just touches the (nonsupporting) rubber mat, with your thighs parallel to the floor, knees slightly in front of your toes, and butt slightly behind your heels (count three). If you are unable to support yourself in this position or you feel in jeopardy of falling, do this exercise for a few weeks directly over a stool or chair, which can be a

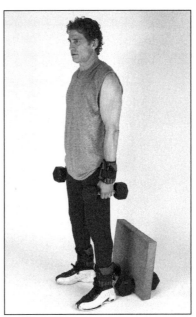

Start position

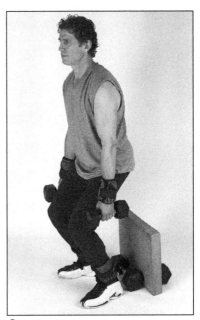

Count one

safety net if you unexpectedly lose your balance.

5. Now, thrust upward back to the standing start position, all the while keeping your head forward, back straight (and arms out in front of you if you're not holding weights as pictured) (count four). Count out as you repeat 12 times, or as many as possible. This is one of the basic push-pull exercises that you may not be able to repeat 12 times initially, even if you're not holding barbells, because your body weight may be more than you can handle.

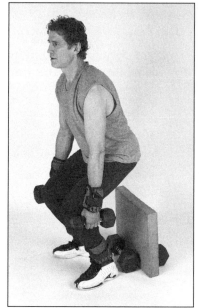

Count two

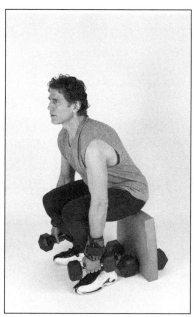

Count three

Exercise 12: Knee Pull (Butt Kick)

1. Start position: Stand with feet shoulder-width apart, hands at sides.
2. Flex your right knee and raise your right heel, aiming for the right side of your right butt (count one).
3. Slowly lower your foot (count two). For this exercise, lowering slowly is actually quite difficult! (Stand near a chair or wall if your balance is questionable, but don't hold on unless you temporarily lose balance.)
4. Continue slowly lowering your foot to the floor (count three).
5. Foot back on floor in starting position (end of count four).

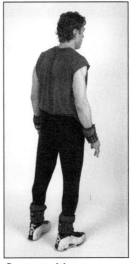

Start position

Repeat steps 1 through 4 using your left leg. Continue to alternate between left and right legs as you count out 12 reps with each leg.

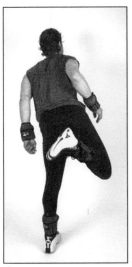

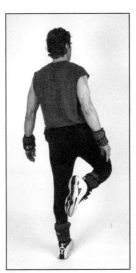

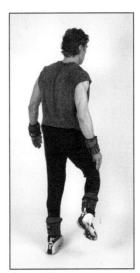

Count one   Count two   Count three

Elbow Push-Pulls: Exercises 13 and 14

The mythic biceps that men, more often than women, stare at are over-rated. For the record, the elbow push-pulls have already been pretty well represented in the multi-joint exercises that you've just completed, but it's an inside joke in the fitness industry that weight lifters of all experience levels get irate if the strength coach dares to omit "mirror muscle" exercises. I'm certainly not going to make that mistake. So assume the position. Yes, your arms will be ripped.

Exercise 13: Elbow Push (Tricep Press)

Pick up slightly lighter dumbbells—you won't be able to lift as much weight with your triceps as you can with your biceps.

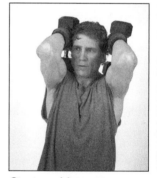

Start position

1. Start position: Hold dumbbells behind neck, with elbows pointing straight forward, forearms parallel to each other.
2. Lift dumbbells straight up, palms facing each other, and hold for a beat (count one).
3. Slowly lower the weights, keeping the upper arms and biceps in tight next to your cheeks (count two).
4. Continue slow descent (count three).
5. Return to start position. The instant the elbow is fully flexed or you feel the dumbbell touch your shoulder (the end of count four), pop the dumbbells up in the air again and repeat the exercise. Count out as you repeat 12 times.

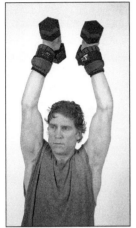

2. Count one

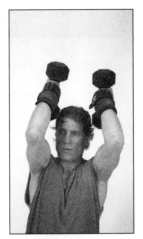

3. Count two

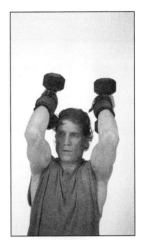

4. Count three

Exercise 14: Elbow Pull (Curl)

1. Start position: Hold dumbbells at your sides, palms facing in, arms straight.
2. Raise the weights: Bend your elbows, raising the dumbbells naturally until elbows are fully flexed, palms adjacent to your shoulders (count one).
3. Slowly lower dumbbells (count two).
4. Continue slow descent (count three).
5. Biceps fully stretched, back to start position (count four). Count out curl 12 times.

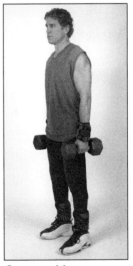

Start position

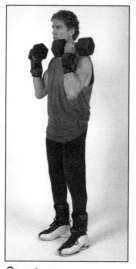 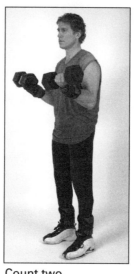 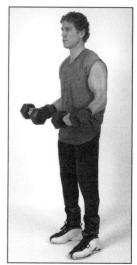

| Count one | Count two | Count three |

Ankle Push-Pulls: Exercises 15 and 16

Ankle exercises are the forgotten stepsisters of circuit training. Ankle push-pulls are vital for women (and cowboys) who wear high-heeled shoes, thereby tightening their calf-Achilles complex, setting the stage for future calf strains when working out in flat tennis shoes. Ankle push-pulls are also key for athletes interested in leg strength, speed, and jumping ability. Most importantly, for our purposes, ankle push-pulls pre-hab foot, ankle, and shin tissues before wear-and-tear damage occurs. And I speak from experience when I tell you that these are the nagging injuries obese exercisers tend to get. Take these exercises slowly; they seem easy, but decades of neglect can't be corrected overnight.

Exercise 15: Ankle Push (Heels Up)

1. Start position: Toes positioned up on the grips of hexagonal 5-pound weights (the heavier the weight, the higher the handgrip, the "harder" the heel lift). Have ankle and wrist weights on and

146

if able hold a moderately heavy dumbbell in one hand.

2. Ankle push: Elevate your heels all the way up until you're standing on your tiptoes on the dumbbell hand grip (count one). Hold on to a nearby wall or chair initially; soon you should be able to balance with minimal or no support.

3. Slow descent (count two).

4. Continued slow descent (count three).

5. Calves are stretched; heels are back down on floor, in start position (count four).

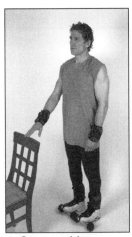

1. Start position

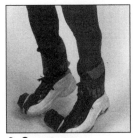

2. Count one

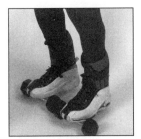

3. Count two

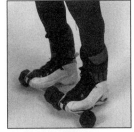

4. Count three

Repeat ankle pushes with following counts: 2–2-3-4, 3–2-3-4, etc., for 12 reps of about 4 seconds each.

Exercise 16: Ankle Pull (Toes Up)

1. Start position: Now heels are on a 5-pound handgrip, toes angled down, one hand on the back of chair (or wall) for support. Women, start out by draping one 10-pound weight on your rubberized mat; men, two 10-pound weights. As shown, place a 20-pound weight at the bottom of the rubber mat to keep the mat and weights from sliding off of the top of your foot. Increase the amount of weight on the mat—which you will be lifting with your toes—as soon as it's

evident that your shin muscles can handle more (when/if you're not sore at all the next day).

2. Ankle pull: Raise your toes up as high as they'll go, lifting the mat with weights (count one).
3. Slow descent (count two).
4. Continued slow descent (count three).
5. Back to start position with shins stretched (count four).

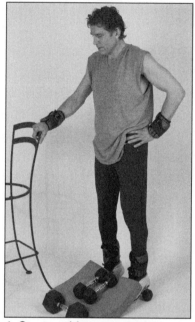

1. Start position

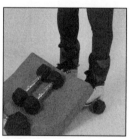

2. Count one

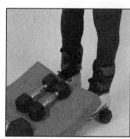

3. Count two

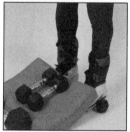

4. Count three

Repeat ankle pulls, counting out 12 reps of about 4 seconds each.

In month two, we'll add twist and balance elements, and when that's mastered, we'll start ramping up the resistance.

PPT TRAINING—STEP-BY-STEP—MONTH TWO

Adding Twist and Balance Components

The balance elements can easily be tacked onto every standing exercise. This is illustrated in figures 1 through 6:

- You can hold dumbbells and lift them while sitting in a chair (figure 1), but to burn more calories and get total body agility and balance benefits, it pays to make the exercise more difficult by:
- Doing the exercise standing up (figure 2).
- Doing the exercise with most of your weight shifted onto one foot. (figure 3).
- Doing the exercise standing on one foot (toes of the other foot just off the ground to stabilize yourself in case you lose your balance) (figure 4).

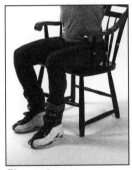
Figure 1

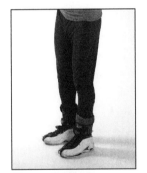
Figure 2

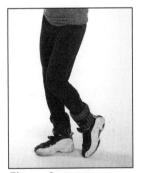
Figure 3

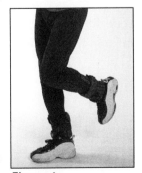
Figure 4

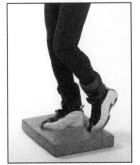
Figure 5

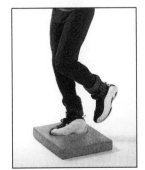
Figure 6

- Doing the exercise standing first with most and then all of your weight on one foot on an unsteady surface (the rubber mat), toes of the other foot just off the mat to stabilize yourself in case you lose your balance (figures 5 and 6).

The next time you trip on an uprooted sidewalk slab, you'll now have a fighting chance. Specific instructions for adding twist and balance elements to each of the 16 exercises beginning in month two follow:

Exercise 1: Top Shoulder Push (Military Press) with Added Twist and Balance Component

1. As before, stand holding dumbbells at shoulder height, just to the outside of each shoulder, palms facing forward with elbows fully flexed below your wrists. Now, transform the military press into a total body workout, stand only on your slightly bent right leg—with your left toes just touching the floor out behind for support.
2. Push dumbbells directly upward, twisting your palms from facing front to facing toward each other as your arms fully extend overhead (count one).
3. Slowly lower (count two).
4. Continue to slowly lower (count three).
5. Back to start position (count four).

On the subsequent lift, twist your palms from facing front to facing toward the outside. Count out 2–2-3-4, 3–2-3-4, 4–2-3-4, etc., as you repeat in-and-out hand twists while doing top shoulder pushes. On the sixth rep, switch from standing on your right leg to standing on your left leg and continue the previous steps for 6 reps.

Exercise 2: Top Shoulder Pull (Chin-Up)

This exercise has no twist or balance maneuvers; therefore, perform it as before.

Exercise 3: Waist Push (Reverse Sit-Up)

This exercise is a reverse sit-up with an added twist element.

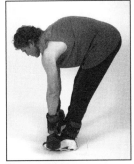

Count three

1. Start position, counts one and two remain the same. Keeping knees straight, bend forward at the hips, allowing barbells to slowly lower toward the top of your feet. Pull your shoulders back to maintain proper position if you tend to hunch. Once you have flexed forward all the way (over three seconds—the same as for the standard reverse sit-up), don't pause or bounce at the bottom of the exercise when barbells are over shoelaces (count three). Add the twist by lifting up your left shoulder toward the sky, leaving the right shoulder and arm lagging behind—these are done quickly, not full counts (counts four (a) and four (b)).

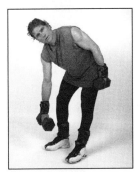

Count four (a)

2. When you're fully standing up (the fourth count), if your feet are facing north, now your upper chest and face should be facing west.

3. Slowly flex forward again until the barbells are over the top of the feet. This time, alternate the movement to the opposite side, lifting up the right shoulder toward the sky, leaving the left shoulder and arm lagging behind.

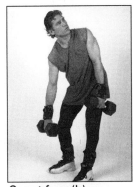

Count four (b)

4. Now do a straight reverse sit-up. Proceed in this manner through a total of 12 reps.

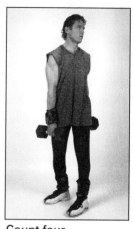

Count four

Exercise 4: Waist Pull (Sit-Up)

These are sit-ups with an added twist element.

1. Assume same start position as original exercise. In a controlled, fluid motion, rise up 60 degrees, pointing the right shoulder toward the left knee (count one). The arms can be in any position—at side (easiest), folded over chest, hands cupped over the ears, arms up extended overhead, or holding a dumbbell or speedball on top of head (most difficult). Don't twist only at the top of the sit-up movement, but perform a controlled twistin motion from the beginning.

2. Slowly lower yourself back down (counts two, three, and four).

3. Do a regular straightforward sit-up.

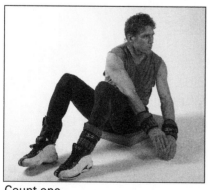

Count one

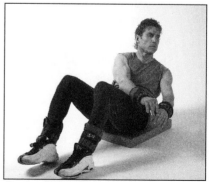

Count two

4. During the next sit-up, aim your left shoulder at your right knee and do the sit-up with twist to the opposite side.

Exercise 5: Front Shoulder Push (Swiss Ball Bench) with Added Twist

Now make an effort to perform your Swiss ball dumbbell bench presses with the added abdominal "plank."

1. Position your shoulders squarely on the Swiss ball, firming your abdomen and back into a firm abdominal "plank" (see photo three on page 133).
2. As you begin the dumbbell bench-press lift, your palms face down toward your feet. Now turn the palms in toward each other as you press up the dumbbells.
3. Slowly descend over the next three seconds to the start arm and hand position.
4. On the subsequent bench press, rotate your palms slightly away from the body (about 30 degrees toward the outside) as you perform the bench press.

Alternate your palms in and palms out as you proceed through 12 reps.

Exercise 6: Front Shoulder Pull (Reverse Ball Bench) with Added Twist

1. As you begin the dumbbell reverse bench, your palms face down toward the feet.
2. Now turn the palms in toward each other as you pull up the dumbbells.
3. Slowly descend over the next three seconds to the starting arm and hand position.
4. On the subsequent bench press, rotate your palms slightly away from the body (about 30 degrees toward the outside) as you perform the reverse bench.

Alternate your palm positions as you proceed through 12 reps.

Exercise 7: Hip/Buttock Push (Donkey Kick)

There are no balance or twist adjustments for this exercise. However, for the month-two adjustment, use your new strength to increase your ankle weights and hold your thigh in the parallel-to-the-ground position for an extra second. Do the 12 reps on each side.

Exercise 8: Hip/Buttock Pull (Knee Up) (Marching Band Leader) with Added Twist

1. Start position: stand comfortably near a wall or chair for safety, feet shoulder-width apart, elbows bent at 90 degrees, but don't grab hold unless your balance feels iffy.
2. Bend your left leg upward at the hip joint (let the calf fall down limply) and twist your left knee outward and up, touching your hand (count one).
3. Slowly lower your left thigh back down (counts two and three). This is difficult.

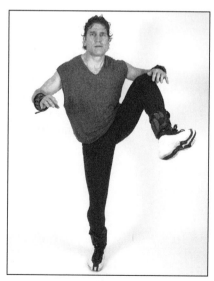 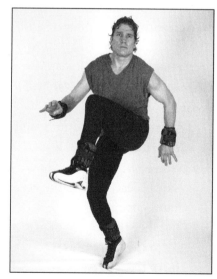

Count one (Outside Hip Twist)   Count one (Inside Hip Twist)

4. Temporarily touch the left foot down on the floor to the start position (count four).
5. Now bend your left hip joint upward and inward, aiming the left knee to your right palm (count one).
6. Again, slowly lower your left thigh back down (counts two and three).
7. Return to the start position (count four). Now proceed through the knee-ups with the inside and outside hip twists with the right leg.

Alternate legs as you perform 12 reps with each leg.

Exercise 9: Side Shoulder Push (Angel Wing) with Added Twist and Balance Component

Perform the exercise first on your right foot (6 reps), then left foot (6 reps).

1. As you begin the up angel wing, your palms face your thighs.
2. Now rotate the palms frontward as you raise your outstretched arms.
3. Slowly lower your arms during the next three seconds while returning to the start arm and hand position.
4. On the subsequent up angel wing, rotate your palms 45 degrees toward the back.

Alternate palm positions while performing 12 reps.

Exercise 10: Side Shoulder Pull (Reverse Angel Wing) with Added Twist

1. As you begin the reverse angel wing, tugging down against the resistance of your bands, your palms face down toward the floor. Turn the palms forward as you execute the lift.
2. Slowly allow your arms to be tugged upward during the next three seconds as you return to the start arm and hand position.
3. On the subsequent reverse angel wing, rotate your palms 30 degrees toward your backside.

Alternate palm positions as you proceed through 12 reps.

Exercise 11: Knee Push ("Mat" Squat)

This exercise has no twist or balance elements. For the month-two adjustment, use your increased flexibility to squat a bit deeper. You've been touching your butt down on the highest edge of the mat, about 20 inches off the ground, now set the mat on its other side, which is closer to 16 inches high.

Exercise 12: Knee Pull (Butt Kick) with Added Twist

Instead of doing straight-up butt kicks (right heel to right buttock) as before, you'll now kick outward, then inward for a total of 12 repetitions each side to better work the hamstrings. Stay with moderate ankle weights.

1. Start position; knee is straight.
2. Let your arms hang comfortably by your sides. Now flex the right knee outward, aiming for your right palm (outward twist)(count one).
3. Slowly lower foot (count two).
4. Continue slowly lowering foot toward the floor (count three)— stand near a chair or wall for safety, but don't hold on unless you temporarily lose balance.
5. Back to start position, foot on floor (count four).
6. Immediately proceed to inward butt kick. Flex the right knee again, but this time aim your heel inward toward the left side of your left butt (inward

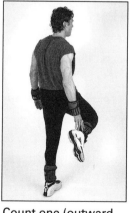

Count one (outward butt kick)

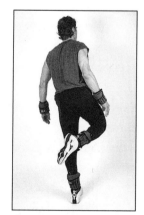

Count one (inward butt kick)

twist)(count one).
7. Again slowly lower foot (count two).
8. Continue to slowly lower foot to the floor (count three).
9. Back to start position for an instant only (count four). Now alternate to the left leg.

Perform 6 inward and 6 outward butt kicks with each leg.

Exercise 13: Elbow Push (Tricep Press) with Added Twist and Balance Element
1. Perform the exercise while standing balanced on one leg, first your right (6 reps), then your left leg (6 reps).
2. As you begin the curl, your palm is facing up toward the sky. Complete the exercise.
3. When you begin the next repetition, rotate your wrist as you raise the weight in until the palm is facing down toward the floor at the top of the curl.

Alternate palm positions as you perform 12 reps (6 on right leg, 6 on the left).

Exercise 14: Elbow Pull (Curl) with Added Balance Component
Perform exercise while standing balanced on one leg, first on right (6 reps), then on the left (6 reps). Otherwise, perform this exercise exactly as previously described.

Exercise 15: Ankle Push (Heels Up) with Added Twist
Advance to doing both ankle push and pull exercises with your feet resting on the hand grips of the 15-pound hexagonal dumbbells for slightly greater stretch.
1. Try the first 6 repetitions with a subtle twist: while performing the heel lift, transfer most of your weight to the small-toe side of your

foot (the big toes feel like they're coming off of the dumbbell grip just a whisker). Your toes still point straight and forward; knees remain fixed (don't let knees go bowlegged).

2. Perform the second 6 repetitions with an opposite twist: with the little toes off of the dumbbell grip just a whisker. Your toes still point forward, and knees remain fixed (not knock-kneed).

Exercise 16: Ankle Pull (Toes Up) with Added Twist

1. Try the first 6 repetitions with a subtle twist: while performing the toe raise, emphasize the big-toe side of the foot being a little higher than the small-toes side. Your feet still point straight and forward; knees remain fixed (don't let knees go bowlegged).
2. Perform the second 6 repetitions with an opposite twist: raise the toes emphasizing the little-toe side of the foot, feet still pointing straight and forward, knees remaining fixed (not knock-kneed).

PUSH-PULL-TWIST TRAINING—STEP-BY-STEP— MONTH THREE AND BEYOND

- Stay with the original PPT philosophy.
- Now progress to two sets of 12 repetitions for each exercise.
- As before, start with the one set of the push exercise, followed by one set of the pull exercise, then repeat another set of the same push then pull exercises.
- If you're not able to do both sets of 12 repetitions, the weight is too heavy. If you could still do two to three more reps, the weight is too light.
- Initially, you're going to have to write down the weight amounts you use during each exercise session, as regular adjustments will have to be made to perfect the resistance settings.
- Contract muscles a little quicker on ascent (the hard part of lift).
- Slow down the easy (eccentric) part of the lift, perhaps to four seconds.
- Never increase the resistance, sets, reps, or the speed of a lift if muscle soreness persists. And keep in mind: Soreness may peak 48

to 72 hours after a particular exercise session.
- Never do "max" lifting (a weight you may or may not be able to lift off the rack) at this stage of your weightlifting program.
- Combine single-joint moves into unique multi-joint exercises to spice up your strength workouts.

Get your family and friends involved!

The WOW! ℞ Motivation/Inspiration Follow-Through

It is important to follow through with these actions:

- Write in your thought journal both sabotaging thoughts and mental or physical "wins." This may be easiest to do alongside your food and exercise journals rather than separately.
- Weigh yourself each Monday morning and record it in your journal—to visualize your progress, create a graph of your results using an Excel spreadsheet or other graphing program.
- Track your week-by-week progress alongside *The Biggest Loser* 36 states "Home" contestants (but compare only your percentage weight loss, not absolute pounds lost. Some on-air contestants, understandably, drank extra fluid to artificially inflate their first week's weigh-in and some TV weeks were really 10 or more days. Additionally, despite intense efforts by NBC, the show producers, and myself, some participants, ill-advisedly, dehydrated to further affect results [short-term "help," long-term detriment to weight loss]).
- Congratulate yourself! You're doing it! Share the results of your progress with your "fat-fighter" support team. Week after week you've found ways to succeed despite business lunches, family outings organized around meals, personal health issues, financial costs, moments of waning motivation, bad weather, and the

rest of "life." But you've prevailed; you're doing the work to reach your WOW! weight! When you hit it—and you will—learn and master The WOW! ℞ obesity survivor's maintenance manual (page 270), and keep the fat off forever!

That is it—the big secret! The novel program that *The Biggest Loser* at-home contestants followed to lose over 25 percent of their starting weights—essentially all fat—without time off from their busy lives at home and at work, without trainers, food services, or Internet diet pills. Rather than eating a little less and having their motivation evaporate when less-than-desired physical change was apparent; rather than eating a lot less and—since no diet works long term—down the road having their appetites return and, soon, all the lost weight boomerang back on, the home contestants ate a little less and exercised a lot more. Their fat came off, literally, day by day. The qualities and quantities of food they ate kept hunger at bay. The exercise—unlike a "diet," which the subconscious brain fights tooth and nail—became routine. Even in the face of dramatic weight loss, this level of exercise, on average, grew muscle—something never before seen with any weight-loss pill, diet, or surgery! Plus, the exercise kept the daily calorie burn high and brain feel-good chemicals pumping; it accelerated the achievement of WOW! weight and, most importantly, it put them in the very best possible position to maintain fat loss permanently. Sound simple? It is! That's the beauty of this home-based, no-gimmick, no-pills, nonsurgical, and all regular store-bought food, fat-loss program.

But believe me, simple doesn't always mean easy, especially if you get an orthopedic ding and have to find nonirritating exercises that keep up the calorie burning and body reshaping while allowing your injury to heal. Sometimes, when you come home from a stressful making-a-living day without fattening comfort foods to drown your sorrows, your head hurts more than your achy muscles and joints. You'll relate to the psychological pitfalls the contestants experienced and benefit from advice they were given by weight-loss psychologists.

Whether you're obese or morbidly obese and want to lose impressive amounts of fat quickly and safely, or prefer to lose excess fat somewhat more gradually, or if you're overweight and need to lose fewer pounds of fat, this at-home fat-loss program takes you step-by-step through the process.

SECTION TWO

YOU ARE NOT ALONE

Follow the Losers

Chapter Nine

The WOW! ℞: Week-by-Week Guide

COMPARE YOUR PROGRESS TO THE AT-HOME
BIGGEST LOSER PARTICIPANTS

I'm hoping this section will be the highlight of the book for you. Previous popular diet books have offered specific reduction plans, but prior to this, none have ever scientifically tracked the true response of a large group of obese subjects who lived the books' recommendations at home. This section is real time with real emotions; it chronicles the behind-the-scenes weight-loss struggles and triumphs of 36 everyday people with families and hectic schedules and excess fat—just like you—who finally decided to put their health first.

Day One: *Doctor Motivation Speech*
"Hello, I'm Doc H., good to see you all again. For the last several weeks, each one of you has been on an emotional roller coaster. First, you're up, TV producers are flying you out to L.A.—you made the show. Right? Then you see all the other folks at the medical exams and think: No way, there's too much competition; I can't possibly make it. Next you get shuttled to the ranch, where makeup artists and hair stylists prep you for your photo shoots and you think: Hey, maybe I made it!

Tonight you weren't selected—you didn't make the show. You're feeling miserable."

I was not real happy either. The entire group was silent and sullen—not the bubbly, gregarious folks I'd examined just a week before. I knew many of these rejected contestants were stress eaters, alcoholics, or had issues with depression, anxiety, abandonment, and trust. Was a breakdown inevitable? Was this rejection going to trigger a binge of late-night whoppers. . . or some other fast-food entrée?

"But wait, there's one more twist. I'm here to tell you: You have been chosen! You won't be seen much, if at all, on TV, but from my vantage point, you've been chosen to act in perhaps the most meaningful TV role of all time. You see, right now obesity researchers laugh off *The Biggest Loser* show. They don't believe it has even one snit of relevance to 160 million overweight and obese Americans. Weight-loss doctors have acknowledged—and I guarantee you—that each TV contestant will lose a king-sized chunk of fat, but the obesity researchers wave this off as a "weight-loss fantasy." They write medical journal editorials calling what takes place on the ranch a "Pollyanna world"—and, you know, maybe that's true. The 14 people chosen today for the TV show will be isolated on the ranch, away from all their work pressures, and will have at their disposal all sorts of assistance.

"Still, all of you—representing 36 states and all walks of life—have been chosen to see if obese individuals can achieve dramatic weight loss at home on their own with no ranch "accoutrements"—just an intensive three-day hands-on seminar on exercise, healthy eating, and weight-loss psychology. Then it's all you. You go back home to your families and jobs. You take responsibility and self-start The WOW! ℞—with no fancy equipment, trainers, or food services. You will e-mail in your Monday morning weight and participate in an hour group support call Monday P.M. We'll work as a team—encouraging sister-state members, rather than stabbing each other in the back to advance toward a statistically unobtainable pot of gold.

"Here's why the 'you're chosen to act in perhaps the most meaningful TV role of all time' line isn't bogus Madison Avenue hype. We are going to burn off your fat while you continue your normal daily routines and responsibilities at home without wheelbarrows of prize money being pushed in front of your noses. And if you lose your excess fat, if you get healthy, if you extend your life—then so can the other 160 million overweight and obese Americans! Are you up for the task?

"Number one, stand up, because you burn 33 percent more calories when you're standing, compared with sitting. Number two: I want you all to hold hands while I introduce you to yourselves, the group chosen to make a difference, to spearhead the drive against the obesity epidemic. Averaged out, you are 32 years old; you have 110 pounds of excess fat. The majority of you are prediabetic, hypertensive, and hyperlipidemic, right on track to die young. You all have excuses. I heard almost every excuse imaginable when I spoke with you individually: You can't work out 'cause it's too cold (my nose hairs freeze), too hot, too rainy, no time, too much time, too self-conscious, too tired, too achy, a past back problem. . . . You've been on 'diets' before; you've all played psychological head games with yourselves.

"Before your bus arrived here from the ranch, I was pacing outside, feeling a weird kind of energy. I flashed back 20-some years ago when I was standing in the Tampa locker room before our Raiders–Redskins Super Bowl game. The crowd in the stadium above was stomping so hard that the concrete girders were vibrating. I was huddled with a group of players in the training room, nervous as can be, when Coach Flores walked in, calm as a cucumber.

"I'll never forget it. He called the team together and said, 'Men, stay with the basics. Don't try to out-fancy your opponent. Your talent will prevail.'

"We won that game, by the way.

"So, I stand here today and instruct you: *Stay with the basics.*

- Adopt a regular schedule of sleep, meals, and exercise.
- Journal your daily food and exercise calories.
- Stay with fresh fruit, vegetables, skim milk, soy, and other lean protein from fish, chicken, and turkey. Consume good fats and whole grains. Eat red meat sparingly.
- Exercise intensely at the same times each day—an hour each morning and each afternoon, six days a week.

"Don't 'out-fancy' yourself.

- You don't need fake food with artificial fats and sugars.
- You don't need "weight-loss potions." The one severe medical complication I've seen doctoring for this show was after a contestant took an over-the-counter weight-loss tea.
- You don't need complicated exercise machines or heart monitors.
- Don't dehydrate, salt deplete, or carb deplete. There's no shortcut to your "WOW!"—With-Out-Waist—weight.

"If you follow The WOW! ℞, I guarantee you'll win energy, you'll win health, and you'll win life! Tomorrow morning you'll take the first steps together at 5:30 A.M. sharp, our first exercise class. And when the sun comes up, and you're walk-jogging by the Manhattan Beach lifeguard

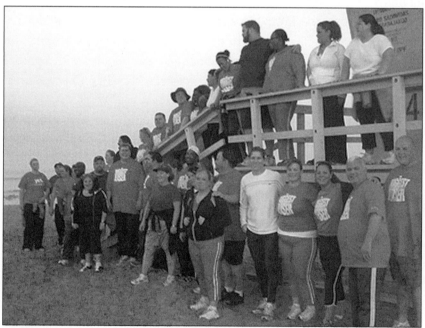

Surrounded by my 36 State Home Team after the first half of our initial 5-mile walk/jog... some did well, some needed to ride partway in a back-up van.

stations, the ocean breeze in your lungs, it'll sink in. You have been chosen! Up to this moment, you're a loser. But now, it's winning time!"

During the next three days, our team taught the 36, now called the *36 State Home Team*, everything they needed to know about the basics of The WOW! ℞—the same information contained in this book—and put them through some preliminary paces. I told them where to e-mail their weekly weights and sent them home to begin my program on their own turf.

Now I'll give you a week-by-week peek into the same program the 36 State Home Team followed, sharing with you the behind-the-scenes challenges they encountered and the secrets of their tremendous fat-loss success! And I guarantee that as you participate and follow along on the program, you won't feel alone, but part of a team of millions of other Americans courageously stepping forward to change their lives forever—by losing excess fat while maintaining or even gaining bone and muscle mass, and achieving better health.

It's time to get back into your "thin" clothes—and your life!

THE WOW! ℞—DAY ONE

Fat-Loss Preparation Checklist

- On day one, before you begin:

  - Be sure to see your physician for a pre-participation examination and screening to assure that your current health status is adequate to embark on this program of caloric restriction and up to two hours of exercise a day.
  - Take the Home Depression Screen (see Section Three) and consult a qualified licensed therapist, if need be.

- Obtain your body-fat percentage measurement—preferably via Bod Pod, underwater weighing, iDEXA, or DEXA. (If such body-fat testing is not available in your area or the cost is beyond your budget, refer to Chapter Six for alternative methods to estimate your body-fat percentage.)

• Compile your "home" baseline body composition data (see Chapter Five for details) to include:

- Weight first thing on Monday morning.
- Measurement of your waist circumference (parallel to the floor at level of belly button after the end of breath out).
- Photos taken of your whole body, wearing a bathing suit (two-piece for women), from the front, side, and back at exactly six feet away. Retake the pictures each month.
- Goal clothes: Select an outfit you'd like to fit into when you reach your WOW! weight.

• See instructions in Chapter Five to calculate:

- Your resting daily energy expenditure (RDEE).
- Your individualized minimum calories per day (RDEE $\times$ 0.8).

If you become tired, lethargic, or repeatedly hungry, automatically increase your daily calorie allotment to your full RDEE and take off a day from exercising. If that doesn't work, consult with the physician that you've appointed to head up your health team.

- Your WOW! weight (ideal weight).

• Set up your journals (samples in appendix)—either in a notebook you'll continue to use to track your progress or on a computer spreadsheet—to include these items:

- Exercise
- Food
- Thoughts

- Exercise equipment to have on hand:

  - Home gym (see list of items in Chapter Eight)
  - Running gear
  - Reusable ice bags (bags of frozen peas work just as well)

- Calorie-counting tools to have on hand:

  - Calorie-counting book
  - Kitchen food scale
  - Cooking-oil misters
  - Meal planner (see Section Three)

- Finish lacing your running shoes. You're ready to start!

THE WOW! ℞—WEEK ONE

Begin Week-One Agenda— Daily Routine

The morning routine includes the following:

- Dynamic warm-up and outdoor brisk walk-jog away from home for 30 minutes, then turning around and heading back, aiming for 4.5 to 5 miles (make sure you've gone at least 4 miles).
- Immediate post-exercise anabolic shake or carb-protein snack ($1/12$ of daily calorie allotment).
- A multimineral/multivitamin with calcium (500 mg, men; 1,000 mg, women) and vitamin D (400 IU).

- Morning snack ($^1/_{12}$ of daily calorie allotment).
- Lunch ($^1/_4$ of daily calorie allotment).
- Afternoon snack ($^1/_{12}$ of daily calorie allotment).

The afternoon/evening workout includes:

- Monday, Wednesday, and Friday: one-half hour of aerobics, then one-half hour of Push-Pull-Twist training.
- Tuesday and Thursday: one hour of recreational sports or aerobics.
- Saturday (or Sunday): two- to three-hour nature hike or active family outing.
- Immediate post-exercise anabolic shake or carb-protein snack ($^1/_{12}$ of daily calorie allotment).
- Dinner ($^1/_4$ of daily calorie allotment).
- Completing your exercise and food journals and tally totals.
- End-of-day snack—avoid carbonation, fat, acid, caffeine, or alcohol ($^1/_{12}$ of daily calorie allotment).
- Writing in your thought journal.
- Getting a good night's sleep.

The end-of-week routine includes:

- Weighing yourself first thing Monday morning.
- Calculating your weight-loss percentage (pounds you lost the prior week divided by your original weight).
- Tallying your average week's calories consumed (add up each day's calorie intake and divide by seven).
- Tallying your total week's exercise hours (vigorous, moderate endurance, and circuit weightlifting).
- Reviewing your thought journal.
- Reading Dr. H.'s weekly recap.

- Comparing your weight-loss numbers and your trials and tribulations with the 36 State Home participants at same stage of the program.

Dr. Huizenga's Recap—Week One

"What? You're Going to Take Me Out Again?"

Day Seven, 5:20 A.M. e-mail to the 36 State Home contestants:

You're actually doing it!!! This thought journal entry says it all— "My shell-shocked dogs are staring up at me this morning as I put on my tennis shoes yet again as if to say, 'What? You're going to take me out again?'"

Since we've started all this exercise, lots of you are bothered by muscle and joint aches; generalized knee pain seems to be at the top of your complaint list. Guess what? Not much is constructed to handle an extra 100 pounds; just look at our three days together—two broken chairs and a destroyed stair! Your spine, hips, knees, and feet are definitely not meant to carry any overage. I know, because a few years ago, on weekends when I'd hike with my daughter, she'd tire out and I'd jog for a while with her on my back. Almost instantly, carrying the extra 60 pounds, my back and knees, which generally felt great, start absolutely killing me. Many of you constantly carry around twice as much extra weight. I've felt your pain!

Week-One Totals for the 36 State Home Contestants:

Average weight loss: women, 4 pounds; men, 8 pounds
Average weight-loss percentage: women, 1.8%; men, 2.4%

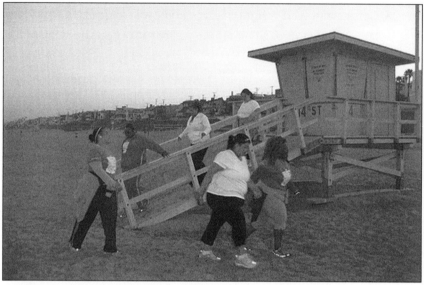

The 36ers had aches and pains...but kept going!

A recommended knee prescription includes:

- Before exercise, ice over the aching side(s) of the knee (an Ace bandage wrapped around a bag(s) of frozen peas or a reusable, formfitting ice pack) for 15 to 20 minutes, and take an anti-inflammatory, such as aspirin, ibuprofen, or naproxen.
- Switch to aerobics with less weight bearing (such as biking, swimming, or elliptical trainer) for one day, then the next day restart the walk-jog or whatever made the knees sore. Continue to alternate days of lower weight-bearing exercise, then higher knee impact. When the pain improves, go back full time to the walk-jog.
- If the pain persists, walk on a treadmill at a slower pace, but up steeper inclines, or switch entirely to nonweight-bearing exercise (biking, swimming or elliptical trainer).

- At the completion of your exercise session, ice again for 15 to 20 minutes (in the car on the way to the office works well).
- Finally, keep losing fat! Getting the extra weight off is by far the single most important treatment.

Lots of you have noted that you were sleeping more. True, with this exhaustive new exercise, you need more recuperative sleep up front. But I promise, very soon, as you get fit, you'll need less sleep and your nights will improve—you'll sleep sounder and wake up more refreshed. (One sign that the dietary admonitions are sinking in—your teammate who operates a tattoo parlor reported dreaming of tattooing fruit baskets on a long line of customers.)

Many of you are peppering me with e-mails about optimum exercise durations, "to keep up with the folks at the ranch who exercise four to sometimes six hours a day." The WOW! ℞ calls for about one hour of intense exercise two times a day, six days a week. I'll explain in full later. . . but for now, basically with this plan we'll get 80 percent of the fat-loss benefits and avoid essentially all the potentially serious side effects that necessitate my having to monitor the folks at the ranch with weekly blood tests. And with four or more hours of exercise a day comes frequent overuse injuries requiring a full-time physical therapist/athletic trainer to keep them going. . . you at home don't have that backup. Trust me, stay with two, or at most two and a half hours a day.

OK, we'll talk next week. . . time for me to go work out my dogs!

THE WOW! ℞—WEEK TWO

Stay with the Week-One Agenda

- Daily exercise as scheduled.
- Daily healthy eating as scheduled.

- Daily entries in your exercise, food, and thought journals.
- Same end-of-week routine.

At the end of week two, consult with a registered dietitian to review a representative three-day food journal to assess your calorie-counting ability. Your physician can refer you to a dietitian who is very affordable—even in an overpriced area like Beverly Hills, a consultation with a top-notch dietitian can be obtained for $100 an hour. (Get a referral from your doc or go to www.eatright.org to help find a licensed dietitian near you.)

Dr. Huizenga Recap—Week Two

The 36 Home Contestants Pass Notoriously Difficult Second Week with Flying Colors!

"Overwhelmed" pretty much summed up all of your Week-One thought journals. Everybody was stressing. There were ungodly 5 a.m. exercise wake-up calls and occasionally muscles moving past sore to stiff and achy. There were alien outer grocery store aisles, a foreign rainbow of fruits and vegetables needing to be prepped, and planning lists of mandatory meals and snacks. Then there were the food, exercise, and thought journals—plus the strict admonition not to sacrifice a drop of sleep. Whew! And to top off the afternoon, the wise guy coworker or relative, or a backstabbing "friend" who finds it easier to drag you back down than clean up his own act, tries to lure you with a donut or some

---

Week-Two Totals for the 36 State Home Contestants:

Average Week-Two weight loss: women, 4 pounds (1.8%); men, 7 pounds (2.1%)

Average total weight loss: women, 9 pounds (3.6%); men, 15 pounds (4.5%)

---

other sugar-laced landmine. The promised energy and mood bump wasn't instantly evident. Instead, a "can I do it?" performance anxiety reigned. Your thought journals showed some mind-bender temptations—but you were able to spot self-sabotage and snuff it out! By the end of the week, a bit of a routine was established. "Overwhelmed" was replaced, in part, by excitement and anticipation of good health to come.

I said at the start, "To lose weight, take every obstacle one stride at a time." One of you e-mailed me, deflating the air from what I thought at the time was a cool quote by claiming your first obstacle was that your feet, shins, and calves were hurting so much from the initial week of exercise that it was now impossible for you to stride, much less jog! True, in sedentary obese folks, the foot/Achilles tendon/calf/knee complex is susceptible. Mechanical forces from the excessive weight bearing overwhelm the connective tissue limits, frequently causing muscle pulls, inflamed tendon connections, fasciitis, and bursitis. Here are some tips that can help you:

Prevent

Start each workout with the full dynamic stretch (Chapter Seven) and, even if you're rushed, end with at least a static stretch of the foot and calf, which are automatically traumatized by excess weight. Here's how:

1. Go halfway down into a squat, then lean forward, putting your hands on the floor, knees remaining bent, feet and heels remaining flat on the floor two to three feet back. Feel a moderate stretch in your Achilles tendon above the heel for 10 seconds (part a).
2. Then walk your hands forward six inches or so, straighten the knees, and lift your pelvis, keeping the heels flat on the floor (part b). Feel a gentle pull behind the knee and high up in the calves for a 10 count. Finally, go up on your fingertips and "walk" your hands back toward your feet and return to the standing position.

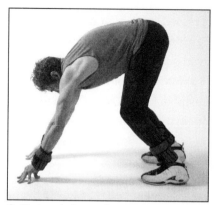
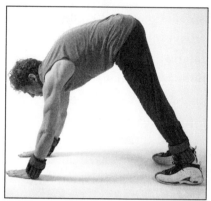

Calf stretch (part a)   Calf stretch (part b)

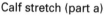

Listen to Your Body

If the pain does not get worse during or immediately after your work-out, then it's okay to continue exercising. If it hurts worse, immediately switch to an activity that's tolerable—for a calf injury, you'd cross-train on a bike, elliptical trainer, or swim, which places less demand on the foot/Achilles tendon/calf/knee system. Swimming effectively works the upper body and core (although all things being equal, swimming re-quires less energy expenditure in the obese because fat causes you to ride up out of the water with less drag forces to overcome), while bik-ing works core and thigh muscles (be sure to use foot clips to work the hip flexors and hamstring muscles, too). Obviously, stay with the anti-inflammatory and ice recommendations I gave in my last letter.

Never Use an Orthopedic Injury as an Excuse to Stop Exercising!

A former contestant proved this point in spades: She suffered a stress fracture of a foot bone, and even though pain prohibited her from run-ning or even walking fast, she still lost 4 or 5 pounds a week! She swam, biked, and used the elliptical trainer while the foot healed and never missed a beat on the weight-loss front.

Completely resting sprains, strains, or tendonitis is an old wives' tale. These painful inflammatory conditions respond better to movement than rest. The outmoded "don't exercise 'til the pain is gone" advice not only delays healing, but also causes collateral damage to the body's metabolism and psyche. Just the other day, I spoke with another former contestant who sorrowfully related that he'd recently gained 25 pounds because he had major shoulder surgery two months prior and was now depressed.

I almost screamed, "What in the world were you thinking? You could have run every day!"

"No way, Doc, you don't understand, when I bounce even a little, the shoulder really kills."

"I do understand," I replied. "I had major shoulder surgery myself a few years ago; the pain's not fun, but you have to keep moving! Find a therapist specializing in athletic rehab! My orthopedist gave me a special sling that secured the shoulder down to my chest, and for more protection against the shoulder moving, I Ace wrapped the heck over that brace, took an over-the-counter anti-inflammatory, then went out running for an hour, 48 hours after surgery."

All in all, I must say the 36 of you passed the notoriously difficult second week with flying colors. Weight loss—but not fat loss—often goes way down in the second week of a diet as the body compensates for first-week fluid and salt losses (yes, first-week weight losses far exceed first-week fat losses). But in spite of these "medical" hurdles, each of you and your 36 home teammates still kicked butt. Remember that first night when we talked about the first step in a long fat-loss journey? Well, we're off to a blazing start. As a team we are right on course to accomplish even the pie-in-the-sky WOW! ℞ weight goals.

For the handful of you who only lost a couple pounds, remember, The WOW! ℞ is about losing fat! If you are putting in the work—the hour each A.M. and P.M.—and sticking to your calorie count, I guarantee you're losing lots of fat; some sedentary individuals gain over 5 pounds of plasma (blood) volume to maximize heart efficiency and protect against dehydration and heat stroke (similar to pregnancy fluid gains) in the first weeks of exercise training. This is a normal, protective, and appropriate body response that may make your scale weight more than you think it should be. Your weight is not important. Your fat weight is what we are going to lower. Weight gain from muscle growth and blood volume expansion is good!

Other Questions from Your 36 State Home Teammates

Question: What do I do if I'm hungry after dinner and I've already met my calorie allotment?

Answer: Have an additional high-fiber carbohydrate (either 50 calories of a fruit or vegetable), plus a one- or two-ounce protein snack, such as tuna packed in water, chicken breast, or a boiled egg. Half the yolk "fat" is the heart-helping kind, and, fortunately, on this fat-loss program, cholesterol is not something we need to worry about. (See Section Three for additional snack suggestions.)

Remember: The WOW! ℞ is not about starving yourself. It's about eating multiple healthy meals consisting of satiating foods and pushing away from the table before you're past full. Interestingly, the majority of the 36ers have reported back that their calorie allotment taken with a heavy dose of high-fiber foods is—surprisingly—more than enough.

Question: What do I do if I'm a few hundred calories short of my calorie-consumption "requirement" late at night and I'm not hungry?

Answer: Fine, go to bed. But have a little of your anabolic shake before your morning workout and a full helping afterward. The real worry is that, in the past, when contestants have consistently gone below calorie limits, their workouts suffered—the net effect being less, not more, weight loss, along with fatigue, occasional nausea, and worrisome blood test changes when the muscles repeatedly run out of fuel.

Question: Are warm-ups needed?

Answer: Just doing the exercise at a slower pace for the first five minutes probably suffices. I like to take a quick, hot shower before my morning run (remember, warm-ups are about increasing body temperature a degree or so). The "dynamic warm-up" actively heats and strengthens the musculature while lubricating the joints. As you start to stride, and even run, in future months, the warm-up takes on added importance in preventing injuries.

Question: I live in the humid South and I've been sweating nonstop with all your exercise! At the grocery store, there is a slew of bottled waters, Smart and Vitamin waters, Propel- and Gatorade-type drinks— what's best for me?

Answer: The perfect "rehydration-energy-electrolyte"-enhanced drink for you depends on:

- the intensity and duration of your planned athletic endeavor.
- climatic conditions (temperature and humidity) and thickness of your clothing.
- your level of conditioning (as you get fit, your sweat rate goes up).
- your level of heat acclimatization (as you adjust to the heat, the concentration of salt in the sweat drops markedly).
- your exercise goals—peak performance vs. general fitness vs. blood pressure reduction vs. weight loss (i.e., if high blood pressure is an issue, it's best to only partially replace salt losses).
- your baseline diet and pre-exercise hydration status (if you're able to pee only a small amount of dark-yellow urine pre-exercise, you are at risk for dehydration).

Table 9.1 Comparison of Rehydration Drinks*

	Smart Water	Water (bottled)	Water (municipal)	Water (soft)	Propel	Vitamin Water	Gatorade	Gatorade Endurance	Skim Milk (lactaid)
Calories	0	0	0	0	10	50	50	50	86
Simple sugar(s) (g)	0	0	0	0	3	13	14	14	12
Protein (g)	0	0	0	0	0	0	0	0	8
Fat (g)	0	0	0	0	0	0	0	0	0
Sodium (mg)	0	0 to 20	10 to 60	68	35	0	110	200	127
Potassium (mg)	trace	0	trace	trace	0	60	30	90	409
Calcium**	trace	0	0	0	0	0	0	0	50%
Vitamin C**	0	0	0	0	10%	40%	0	0	4%
Vitamin E**	0	0	0	0	10%	0	0	0	1%
Niacin**	0	0	0	0	25%	0	0	0	1%
B6**	0	0	0	0	25%	20%	0	0	8%
B12**	0	0	0	0	4%	20%	0	0	39%
Other nutrients	Magnesium				Other B vitamins				Vit. D & others
Price/oz	0.06	0.01 to 0.07	0.00	0.00	0.06	0.07	0.05	0.06	0.07

*For 8-oz serving size

**Percent Daily Values are based on a 2,000-calorie diet

• your tolerance of stomach distention during exercise.

• your sex (women produce less sweat than men for comparable heat-exercise stress).

• cost.

You have no need for electrolyte-sugar drinks with noncompetitive exercise lasting less than an hour in comfortable conditions when you consume adequate salt in your diet. If you exercise outdoors in the early morning and early evening (or indoors), your sweat loss should be less than 1,000 cc an hour and sodium loss less than 1,000 mg an hour with negligible potassium, calcium, and magnesium losses.

First, make sure you're drinking enough liquid. Weigh yourself pre-exercise, then add the number of cups you drink: ($^1/_2$ pound per cup) minus urine losses ($^1/_2$ pound per cup) minus your weight at end of exercise equals your net sweat losses, which shouldn't be greater than 1 to 2 percent of your weight. I recommend you drink water on awakening and immediately pre-exercise and every 15 minutes thereafter, with an anabolic shake within 15 to 30 minutes of the conclusion of your workout.

Second, salt your food for the first three months of the program and consume all the core foods; this will replenish all electrolyte and micronutrient losses. Given the sodium losses in your sweat, it would be stupid to pay extra money for drinks with zero sodium (i.e., Smart water, Vitamin water, or some bottled water). (See Table 9.1.) Furthermore, the vitamins contained in some sports drinks may nauseate exercisers and together with the artificial flavors may tint the urine, thereby invalidating the helpful clinical observation that dark-yellow urine signifies dehydration and pale lemonade-colored urine connotes normal hydration (view online urine color charts at: http://www.owlnet.rice.edu/~hea1103/docs/Am%20I%20Hydrated%20-%20Urine%20Color%20Chart.pdf).

Never overdrink water to the point that you need to urinate multiple times during your workout! Your post-workout weight should never be greater than your pre-workout weight. Out-of-condition people who overdrink water risk life-threatening water intoxication or hyponatremia (low level of blood sodium); excessive bathroom visits producing crystal-clear urine is a warning sign.

For your unfit ranch TV mates who are working out four or more hours per day, occasionally midday in the hot California climate, they sweat up to two to three liters per hour with sodium losses initially as high as 3,000 mg per hour. These contestants are instructed to take multiple shots of diluted baking soda pre-exercise, drink copious amounts of tap water beginning one hour pre-exercise, liberally salt their food and ingest the anabolic shake rich in antioxidants and potassium immediately post-exercise. When contestants deviated from this formula, with the misguided belief salt restriction would help them lose weight, blood sodium levels invariably dropped, injuries increased, and the ability to maximally burn fat decreased.

THE WOW! ℞—WEEK THREE

Stay with the Week-One Agenda

Dr. Huizenga Recap—Week Three

It's Never Too Late to Start an Exercise and Food Journal
During our initial several-day exercise-eating cram session, I talked about the fact that while keeping accurate exercise and food journals is a big commitment (okay, it's a big pain in the butt), it's also a phenomenal educational and motivational tool. It helps prevent exercise and diet procrastination—the idea that you can phone in the exercise today and work out twice as hard tomorrow. . . sorry, that doesn't work.

I quoted data from the first three *Biggest Loser* seasons, showing that contestants who counted calories throughout the course of those shows lost about 27 percent of their weight, compared to 16 percent for those who didn't count calories.

Now, after just over three weeks of our home contestants' outstanding efforts, the same trend seems to be emerging. The women who sent in exercise and food journal data have, on average, lost 5.9 percent of their body weight; the women who aren't sending me that data have lost, on average, 3.7 percent. Similarly, the men who've sent in exercise and food journal data have, on average, lost 6.7 percent of their body weight, while the men who aren't sending the data have lost, on average, 4.6 percent.

Yes, there is a method to my madness!

Week-Three Totals for the 36 State Home Contestants

Average Week-Three weight loss: women, 3 pounds (1.2%); men, 5 pounds (1.5%)

Average total weight loss: women, 12 pounds (4.8%); men, 20 pounds (6.0%)

Questions from the 36 Home Contestants

Question: I feel great! Can I exercise three, four, or even more hours a day, like they do on *The Biggest Loser* ranch?

Answer: Yes, you can, but regardless of how great you may feel, I wouldn't advise it. First off, as you may know, certain professional athletes (such as football players in summer camp two-a-days, marathoners, mountain climbers, dog-sled slushers), laborers, farmers (most notably the Amish, who shun modern "energy-saving" equipment), and military recruits exercise vigorously for four or more hours a day. (A contestant in the Iditarod, the Alaskan dog-sled race, was recently found to be exercising off over 10,000 calories a day!)

Only in the last two years did my *Biggest Loser* research prove, for the first time, that more than the boilerplate exercise recommendation of 20 to 30 minutes of walking or a similar wimpy facsimile three times a week was even possible for sedentary obese and even morbidly obese adults!

But at this stage, none of you are professional athletes, world-class mountaineers, seasoned laborers, or farmers who have adapted to strenuous exercise. And don't forget pacing. Every competitor—and serious dieter—has to master the program he or she is following. This is the first leg of our six-month fat-loss journey. We're only one-half lap into that six-lap race. It's okay to sprint out of the blocks to shake the nervous energy, but then you have to settle into a sustainable pace. The last thing you want to do is go out too fast, burn out, and fade in the middle of the race.

My analysis of prior *Biggest Loser* show participants reveals that excessive exercise (especially if coupled with dehydration) has many more medical, orthopedic, and psychological negatives than positives; oddly enough, four or more hours of exercise may not even be the quickest way to lose fat. I'm looking for a smoother course to maximize your fat loss and future weight maintenance. I'm estimating that working out two hours a day (two and a half maximum) as intensely as you are able, six days per week will get you exactly where you need to be: with essentially all excess storage fat stripped away, with the least risk of burnout and injury.

Question: Can I eat whole-wheat pasta?

Answer: Yes, in moderation. This is not a low-carbohydrate diet. When the "core foods" (see Chapter Six for the essential fruits, vegetables, lean meat, and nonfat dairy products) are accounted for, extra calories remain. Whole grains, (including whole-wheat pasta) are a perfectly acceptable healthy choice to fill the calorie gap, especially when consumed with vegetables (tomato sauce for starters) and lean protein.

Question: What's your opinion of snack bars?

Answer: Snacks are an important part of the WOW! ℞. Snacks between meals help minimize mealtime hunger—remember when Mom screamed at you when you snacked before dinner because she was upset that you weren't going to be hungry for dinner?

Snack bars are convenient, portable, and don't need refrigeration. But it's best to use them only as a backup. Look at the ingredient list—as a rule they're full of corn syrup and sugar, high fructose corn syrup, palm oil, and preservatives. Far preferable are natural protein-carbohydrate snacks I've given you (see Section Three, p. 318-320).

P.S. Don't forget what your mom used to say about snacks. Just do the opposite!

THE WOW! ℞—WEEK FOUR

Stay with the Week-One Agenda

Dr. Huizenga Recap—Week Four

Despite the vast majority of you claiming little or no hunger after consuming your allotted calories, several of you wrote in with food-craving stories, asking, "Is my appetite on the fritz?" or, "If I get a sweet craving, is a diet cola or Splenda okay?" or, "Can I have a small square of really good dark chocolate?"

Appetite is a vital link between calories in and calories out. Unfortunately, no one understands its overlapping components very well.

Overlapping Components of Appetite

Hunger. This word is used in medicine for the plethora of mental (i.e., cravings), chemical (i.e., drugs, alcohol, and marijuana), metabolic (i.e.,

Psychological Corner from Dr. Alexa Altman

We're on a journey. Not surprisingly we're already hitting some emotional turbulence. You have left the "fat world" and begun to enter the "fit world." In the fat world you had a map of the city, a compass that worked, you knew your way around. As unhappy as some of you were, you still knew all the fat-world rules. But now you have left that world—forever. The map of the fit world is different; your fat-world compass does not work, and you get easily confused. Sometimes we all want to go back to familiar surroundings, where we don't get lost. Whenever we lose something—in this case an entire lifestyle—a process of grieving occurs. We cannot lose something without grief. In the coming weeks, you may go through denial, anger, bargaining, and depression before arriving at acceptance. For now, cut yourself some slack and allow yourself to grieve the loss of the fat world.

Remember, you are not alone on this journey. Hopefully, you have already enlisted family and friends. When we met initially at the boot camp, many of you were apprehensive about asking for what you want and need. We observed how easy it is to put others' needs before our own. It seems that many of you are seeking and getting the support you need. I cannot stress how important this shift in behavior will be for your physical and emotional health. I've also noticed that those of you who are not receiving the support you would like from friends and family are reaching out to your 36 home contestants support team. . . and it seems to be helping.

Some of you talked about saboteurs in your life. These individuals are toxic and damaging to your growth and health. If you were in an environment that was toxic, what would you do? Protect yourself! You would put on a great big orange protective spacesuit before getting within 100 feet of toxic material. Why let any of it in? I hear many of you expressing this concept. Go ahead, set limits, or you'll have to put on that ugly orange spacesuit.

hormonal, glucose changes), olfactory, and taste cues promoting eating. One interesting theory: Hunger works just fine to balance calories in versus calories out in active, exercising individuals—the hunger mechanism evolved when we as a primitive species were averaging 20 miles of walking/running a day. However, below some threshold level of activity, hunger can no longer appropriately regulate your desire to eat.

Satiation. Doctors use this word to encompass feelings that govern meal size, which, when tweaked, results in cessation of eating. Satiation often lags 20 minutes behind events going on in the stomach. In other words, you can push away from the table still hungry and feel satiated 20 minutes later, even though you haven't eaten any more food.

Other bodily sensations regulate the intra-meal period of no food intake. Some people can skip breakfast and lunch—no problem; however, they're not properly fueled for exercise and when they finally sit down for dinner, odds are they consume more calories than if they'd had multiple small meals and snacks throughout the day.

Stuff we do know:

- Some people eat when they're not hungry because of stressful events, food or candy sitting under their noses, boredom, or television or computer trance states.
- Falling blood-sugar levels may stimulate hunger in general, but

---

Week-Four Totals for the 36 State Home Contestants:

Average Week-Four weight loss: women, 3 pounds (1.5%); men, 5 pounds (1.7%)

Average total weight loss: women, 15 pounds (6.3%); men, 26 pounds (7.6%)

Average total weight loss (calorie counters): women, 18 pounds; men, 33 pounds

Average total weight loss (noncalorie counters): women, 14 pounds; men, 22 pounds

---

do not appear to stimulate hunger in individuals on calorie-controlled eating plans (that's you at this point).

- The satiation pecking order of macronutrients: Protein and high-fiber carbohydrates are the most filling, followed by low-fiber carbohydrates, then fats (nuts appear to have the highest satiation values in the fat category).

- Solid foods are more satiating than liquids—a really practical fact, since beverages now contribute over 25 percent of the calories Americans consume. Studies with endoscopes show that stretching the stomach with progressively larger balloons results in earlier satiation; however, the body soon becomes tolerant to this "stomach-stretch" trick. This may explain why gulping water to fill up the stomach before or during a meal lowers caloric intake over the short term, but is ineffective as a long-term weight-loss remedy.

Lastly, and in answer to your questions, artificial sugar is okay for now—just try, if you can, to slowly detox off of these products that may be totally okay or may, in fact, have a hidden downside. Basically, I'm not a fan of artificial sugar or fat as they may increase your chance of sliding back into high-sugar or high-fat foods. Dark chocolate—we've all read about its good antioxidants—or, better yet, chocolate skim milk, is okay as a rare reward and as part of your post-workout snack.

Just don't forget to journal your calorie intake!

Questions from the 36 Home Contestants

Question: How are we doing?

Answer: Let me put your progress into perspective. Most large medical weight-reduction diets result in a 5-to-10-percent loss over 6 to 12 months. After only four short weeks, you're already at that point! And maybe only three-quarters of the weight loss in the aforementioned medical studies are fat. Worst of all, 90-plus percent of those subjects gain all their weight back. You know. You've been there, done that.

Yes, the program I've articulated is time consuming, and yes, there will be bumps in the road, but stick with the WOW! ℞ and you can lose gastric bypass levels of fat. Much, much more importantly, by enhancing muscle retention and learning about fat-loss exercise, nutrition, and psychology, you'll increase your chances of permanent fat loss. (Actually, the home contestants have already self-distributed many invaluable e-mail psych lessons to each other, demonstrating the power of a support group.)

Encouraging someone to lose 50 or more pounds without a full understanding of fat-loss exercise, nutrition, and psychology is like dumping a champion rower into a boat without oars. The current will carry the boat backward, regardless of the rower's past accomplishments.

Question: I skipped my period. What gives?

Answer: Yes, weight loss can cause skipped periods, spotting, as well as heavy periods. Your menstrual cycle will return to normal after several months. Of course, to be absolutely safe, every woman with even the remote possibility of pregnancy and an abnormal period cycle should do a urine pregnancy test (at least twice). This exercise-fat loss plan is not appropriate for pregnant women. The nutritional needs of a developing fetus are in many ways unique, which could be compromised by a calorie-controlled diet. As a quick aside, pregnancy is definitely possible during a stringent weight-loss regimen—it's happened already during the show. Fat affects reproductive hormones; obesity acts like a low-level birth control pill. Major weight loss, on the other hand, makes you more fertile.

Question: I received a tearful e-mail (print was visibly smeared on my screen) from a contestant who only lost 1 pound last week, asking

"What happened?" Another contestant reported losing 3.5 to 4 pounds for the week, with good adherence to the fat-loss program, but wondered, "Should I be losing more?"

Answer: First off, based on your entry questionnaires, as a group, you each gained weight over the last several years alone. Just staying the same weight is a lot better! Losing 1 pound is better yet.

Having said that, we're striving for a 1.5 percent weight loss per week over the first two months. So, 3 to 4 pounds, 4 to 6 pounds, and 6 to 8 pounds of fat loss per week for those who initially weighed 200, 300, and 400 pounds, respectively, at the start of program would be more typical.

Here's the problem: Your weight loss doesn't always reflect your fat loss. A few contestants gain muscle, lose fat, and lose only small amounts of weight, but their waist and butt sizes get smaller. One of your teammates lost a relatively small amount on the scale, but simultaneously dropped two pants' sizes. Also, your weight can transiently gyrate up or down 5 to 10 pounds (or maybe more) if you salt food versus avoid salt, drink a ton of water versus dehydrate, or carbohydrate deplete versus take in the full recommended complement of fruits and vegetables. Paradoxically, staying tanked up on salt, water, fruits, vegetables, and the other carbs contained in the anabolic shakes increases the safety and effectiveness of fat loss in the WOW! ℞, even though they all cause "water weight gain." (Yes, some, but not all, women also cyclically gain, then lose, up to 5 extra pounds of water weight on a hormonal basis, which can depress them on the gain side and delude them into thinking their weight-loss efforts are extra effective on the loss side.)

Also, some of you who haven't embraced intense exercise yet aren't burning as many calories up front or after exercise is over (the afterburn), some of you may be compensating for the exercise you do by becoming less active around your apartment or home, and lastly some of you may be genetically slower to respond to exercise (but it will happen, I guarantee it).

Please! Just focus on the exercise and healthy eating plan.

Large amounts of weight loss above the previous rough guidelines can be a warning sign of dehydration or glycogen depletion, so stay alert. Again, as previously mentioned, dehydrating or losing muscle weight will be a disadvantage to your long-term fat-loss and health-enhancement goals.

THE WOW! ℞—WEEK FIVE

Week-Five Agenda

- Increase the intensity of daily exercise (you're starting to get fit now!).
- Progress to second-month PPT training (i.e., add twist and balance components now).
- Maintain same calorie allotment.
- Write daily entries in your exercise, food, and thought journals.
- Continue same end-of-week routine.

Dr. Huizenga Recap—Week Five

Home Contestants' Weekly Weight Loss Matches Ranch Contestants for the First Time!

"Who needs the ranch? Who needs the ranch? Who needs the ranch?" That chant echoed repeatedly off the Los Angeles Memorial Coliseum tunnel walls as the hyperventilating 36 State Home contestants were escorted off the field through a mob of well-wishers after a hard-fought tie with the heavily favored *Biggest Loser* ranch squad of 14 and their ever-present trainers.

"I can do this at home on my freaking own!" one irreverent 36er screamed over the din. She tossed the crowd low-cal portabella mushrooms like a rock star flings guitar picks, then finally slipped into the cordoned-off Coliseum kitchen.

"Who needs some overpriced trainer?" another fumed as, in lieu of autographs, he tattooed yet another fruit basket on the arm of a well-wisher while a teammate confided to the clamoring paparazzi, "Wasn't long ago, I was breaking a step, now I step to break records!"

Hyperbole? Okay, maybe the Coliseum bit is a little over the top, but the group's weight loss this week was a real shocker; edging out your ranch mates' weight-loss stats, if only for a week, is quite a triumph! Who would have predicted it? Our team, with full-time family and job responsibilities, reducing pound for pound with a confined squad single-mindedly working out for over four hours a day, and currently on target to best every nonsurgical weight-loss record!

Now the sobering news: In the last week, while most of the 36 home contestants soldiered onward, a minority had life get in the way of body transformations. Some of you had family health issues or job issues or just slipped off the wagon back to your old television, chip-and-dip stomping grounds. Some have gone underground and are not sending in calorie counts or exercise spread sheets. Don't get left behind! We are first and foremost a team. . . a team that wants all of its members to be healthy, a team that wants to stand by the *Baywatch* lifeguard station again with our arms around one another as one big (thin) happy family, with no regrets.

Yes, Virginia, you can dramatically change body shape and cure high blood pressure, diabetes, reflux, and even asthma in only one month, based on extensive medical evaluations of *Biggest Loser* TV participants!

Week-Five Totals for the 36 State Home Contestants:

Average Week-Five weight loss: women, 3 pounds (1.4%); men, 5 pounds (1.7%)

Average total weight loss: women, 18 pounds (7.6%); men, 31 pounds (9.2%)

Questions from the 36 Home Contestants

Question: I know what a calorie is, by definition. Over the weekend someone told me it's the amount of energy used to increase the temperature of one liter of water 1° Celsius. But I don't understand how that translates into the food we eat and how our bodies use it.

Answer: Your friend's definition is correct (if you want to be really arrogant, simply add: "increase the temperature of one liter of water one degree, from 14.5° to 15.5° Celsius").

If you put a teaspoon of margarine in a sealed compartment within a special device called a bomb calorimeter (it pressurizes oxygen throughout the sample, then sends in a spark to literally blow up the food), the burnt margarine will heat up a surrounding one-liter jacket of ice water to the boiling point (100° Celsius). Therefore, we can conclude that the heat combustion of one teaspoon of margarine is 100 calories. On the other hand, a half-cup of grated carrot, when "exploded" in this manner, will heat up the one-liter jacket of ice water to 24° Celsius, meaning it contains just 24 calories. This is the process by which all food calories are determined.

Fats release about 9.4 calories of heat per gram of tissue (dairy, 9.25; meat and eggs, 9.5), carbohydrates release about 4.2 calories per gram of tissue (glucose, 3.7; vegetables, 4.2), proteins release about 5.7 calories of heat per gram of tissue (eggs and cereal protein, 5.8; vegetable and fruit protein, 5.1). Fats have a much higher heat of combustion than other foods because they possess more energy-rich hydrogen bonds.

But, hey, you asked a science question and nothing is that easy. You need to take the above "bomb" energy values and make two more adjustments. First, it turns out that the body can't fully oxidize the nitrogen-hydrogen component of protein—we urinate out urea (NH_2 $CONH_2$) before exploiting this compound's full energy potential—foregoing about 20 percent of protein's heat combustion. Secondly, not every bit of food you swallow actually makes it into the body, so we need to factor in digestibility. Turns out carbs are around 97 percent absorbed (sugars, 98 percent; vegetables, 95 percent; fruit, 90 percent), fats, 95 percent (animal fats, 95 percent; vegetable fat, 90 percent) and protein, 92 percent (97 percent animal protein, 78 to 85 percent fruit and vegetable protein).

How does this translate to you? I'd like you to be aware of all the assumptions that go into the calorie estimates you see on the side of food containers and packaging. Bottom line: When all the computing is said and done, the average protein contains four calories a gram, the average carb contains four calories a gram, and the average fat contains nine calories a gram. But, depending on the specific food you're talking about, the actual numbers can vary by more than 20 percent! And there may be yet another 20-plus percent variability, depending on when you eat the meal compared to when you exercise!

Further takeaway points: From an energy standpoint, a calorie is a calorie, regardless of the source. For instance, 420 stalks of celery are as "fattening" as 1.5 cups of mayo or eight ounces of salad oil. The obvious difference is that fatty foods contain "dense" calories compared with foods high in fiber and water. It would be almost impossible to consume 420 stalks of celery (or 136 green peppers or 102 whole carrots) in a day, but relatively easy to eat one Double Whopper with cheese, medium fries, and a chocolate shake in a single meal. Remember, although a small amount of fat is essential for life—preferably fat in vegetables, nuts, and fish—per calorie, fatty processed foods are less satiating, have less disease-preventing micronutrients (antioxidants), and often contain poisons (trans fats).

Question: Today I joined a running club—somewhat intimidating—anyway, the slowest running group was a 12-minute pace. I didn't want to go with the walkers, so I ended up running four miles in just over 48 minutes. I felt great after the run! However, right now, three hours later, my legs are throbbing, and I can't figure out how I am going to get in another one-hour workout today. I usually do a spinning class at the gym, but my legs won't move, and I don't know if I can even walk for an hour. . . the only things moving are my fingers (and my bowels, which is the silver lining). Any ideas?

Signed, an ex-400-pounder

Answer: Vigorous exercise is exhilarating, but exhausting. . . welcome to the club!

I can see it now, you returning to California, disembarking from the plane in weightlifting gloves and a singlet (wrestling outfit). . . nothing else. . . just 300 pounds of twisted steel and sex appeal!

All kidding aside, after a barn-burner exercise session like that, make absolutely sure that you drink an anabolic shake. Pick up your second hour of exercise for the day with a nice comfortable walk. It will get the blood flowing and reduce the soreness (this acts essentially like the warm-down world-class long-distance runners do after exhaustive races, speeding muscle recovery by gently washing out lactic acid and other breakdown products). Afterward, if you have time, convince a significant other to massage your legs from the shins and calves on up.

THE WOW! ℞—WEEK SIX

Follow the Week-Five Agenda

Dr. Huizenga Recap—Week Six

Question: How can I best track my shrinking fat?

Answer: Most dieters fanatically follow their weight. True, as you burn off fat, your weight will usually decrease, but beware! Weight loss can be a lousy indicator of fat loss—and that goes double early in a diet.

Remember, body weight = excessive fat + essential fat + lean tissue (water, blood, muscle, bone, heart, liver, kidneys, brain, immune glands, etc.). You want the excessive fat as low as possible, the lean tissue as high as practical. It's the amount of centripetal fat, the ratio of fat to lean and the hydration status, not body weight—or the BMI—that is important. Do you know how many so-called "health" experts don't get this?

Want to be a certified weight-loss specialist? Just commit the following general rules to memory:

• Weight loss from dehydration, muscle, bone, vital organs, or essential fat stores is bad. Essential fat is about the last 5 percent in men, the last 12 to 15 percent in women, so this is not a problem for you—yet. But I guarantee that at the end of this process, we'll have several morbidly obese participants who will, in their zeal for perfection, overshoot their target fat-loss goals and become too thin, even gaunt. Talk about a turnaround.

• Weight gain from lean tissue—muscle growth, bone thickening, and the extra water weight vigorous exercisers need—is good.

• Weight loss from excessive fat stores, together with muscle loss, increases the risk of eventual fat regain. . . but registers as relatively more "weight" loss.

• Weight loss from excessive fat stores, together with muscle gain, gives the best body shape and long-term chance of keeping fat off. . . but registers as more modest "weight" loss.

• Every general rule has exceptions. First, water loss can be a good thing in obese folks whose fat stores are partly responsible for flagrant lower-leg edema (swollen ankles). Second, expanding fat stores are "serviced" by increased intra- and extra-cellular fluid stores—this saltwater "lean tissue" is appropriately "lost" as fat is metabolized.

- Bottom line, when you go on a fat-loss program, the bathroom scale is hardly the last word.

Oh, I almost forgot. You asked how to best track your shrinking fat. Later we'll do a repeat Bod Pod and iDEXA scan. These state-of-the-art tests aren't always perfectly accurate, but they're close. For now, follow your waist measurement. Get your significant other to place a tape measure (the kind tailors favor) around your waist, exactly parallel to the floor, level to your belly button. Take a breath in, and then exhale. At the end of the breath out, take the waist circumference reading. Five to six weeks into The WOW! ℞, I'm looking for a drop in the "umbilical" waist circumference of about 5 percent (about two-thirds of your expected 7 to 8 percent weight-loss percentage). Don't measure your "thinnest" waist, as some doctors mistakenly do, because an obese person's contours change so drastically that at the end of the weight drop you have no idea where to make comparison measurements.

Lastly, any of you like to win sucker bets? Casually ask someone what their waist size is, then, when they tell you, bet them that it's two inches greater than the number they quoted you. Pull out your measuring tape and be prepared to collect (unless they've read this book). Most people assume that their waist size is the same as their pants size, but no one knows his or her true pants size anymore. Every last patient whose waist I measure tells me their pants size is one to four inches less than what I measure. Why this confusion? Vanity tailoring. Today's clothing manufacturers knowingly print incorrect sizes on clothes; if the pants say 34-inch waist, in reality it's closer to 36. Manufacturers understand that the truth could hurt sales. If two pairs of pants fit equally well, people will buy the one with the smaller waist size.

> **Week-Six Totals for the 36 State Home Contestants:**
>
> Average Week-Six weight loss: women, 3 pounds (1.3%); men, 5 pounds (1.7%)
>
> Average total weight loss: women, 21 pounds (8.8%); men, 36 pounds (10.7%)

THE WOW! ℞—WEEK SEVEN

> **Week-Seven Totals for the 36 State Home Contestants:**
>
> Average Week-Seven weight loss: women, 3 pounds (1.3%); men, 4 pounds (1.4%)
>
> Average total weight loss: women, 24 pounds (10.0%); men, 40 pounds (11.9%)

Follow the Week-Five Agenda

Dr. Huizenga Recap—Week Seven

These numbers are truly dramatic. Remember, most studies with Atkins or other popular diets result in only half of this amount of weight lost despite a full year of dieting! We are all in a great position to achieve entirely new bodies at the end of six months. Don't veer from The WOW! ℞ plan. Stay consistent. I know some of you are feeling pressured to do things differently over the short term (i.e, exercise four or more hours a day like the ranch group), but why should you? We're getting fewer muscle and joint injuries, we're adapting better psychologically to the stress of the entire fat-loss process, and we're continuing on with our busy lives while losing close to *Biggest Loser* numbers. It may take longer for some of you to reach the summit, but we will still get to our WOW! weights!

THE WOW! ℞—WEEK EIGHT

Follow the Week-Five Agenda

Dr. Huizenga Recap—Week Eight

"No Retreat, Baby. . . No Surrender."
It was a very interesting week for the home contestants. The announce-ment that weigh-ins would occur to determine who might return to the ranch pumped up stress levels and, I believe, prompted many to in-crease their exercise and shave a few extra calories off their diets. In the face of this (for reasons I'm still trying to fully decipher), the weekly weight-loss amounts of the 36 home contestants (specifically the women) paradoxically decreased compared to previous weeks!

Suffice it to say, the women could have exercised less or eaten a lot more than you reported in your journals; or there may be an exercise-diet "sweet spot" and when you exercise longer or eat less you may unexpectedly burn off less fat, either because the body somehow becomes more energy effi-cient, or exercise becomes less intense, or you become "lazier" and move far less during the nonexercising part of your day. If there is a weight-loss "sweet spot," I'm more convinced than ever that one hour of exercise twice a day, along with moderate caloric intake, is close to the mark.

In terms of comparing yourself to others in our group, women whose weight loss at this point is less than 10 percent (start weight minus cur-rent weight × 100 divided by start weight) or men whose weight loss at this point is less than 12 percent are in the lower half of our group—but don't make any drastic changes. With less than a handful of exceptions, I can see that all of you are working exceptionally hard, with steady im-provement each week. Your weight loss may be a little slower because it takes some people a few extra months to sufficiently reawaken mus-cle before the fat-burning effect of exercise fully manifests itself. Typi-cally, those are people who are a little older and started the program with

> **Week-Eight Totals for the 36 State Home Contestants:**
>
> Average Week-Eight weight loss: women, 1 pound (0.6%); men, 5 pounds (1.7%)
>
> Average total weight loss: women, 26 pounds (10.6%); men, 45 pounds (13.4%)

less muscle and less "athletic" memory. But be assured, good things are happening and great things are about to happen both inside and outside of your bodies.

As you now know, two (not just one as originally promised) of you will return to the ranch in California. Although I wish all of you could have made it back, remember that the ranch has absolutely nothing to do with your long-term goals of achieving optimal health and weight. In fact, competing on the ranch with "weight loss of any type" as your only goal could actually interfere with losing fat and gaining muscle, thus dimming your long-term prospects for weight maintenance... so be careful what you wish for.

It's been a treat watching each of you shrink physically and grow emotionally in front of my eyes. We're almost a third there, DO NOT SLOW DOWN!

"We made a promise we swore we'd always remember,
no retreat, baby... no surrender."
BRUCE SPRINGSTEEN

THE WOW! ℞—WEEK NINE

Week-Nine Agenda

Stay with the same agenda, but with the following changes:

Daily Exercise as Scheduled, with these Adjustments

A.M. Workout: Dynamic warm-up and increasingly intense outdoor jog (now with only occasional walking) away from home for 30 minutes, then turn around and head back, aiming for five miles.

P.M. Workout: On Monday, Wednesday, and Friday, do a 10-minute aerobic warm-up, then 50 minutes of month-three PPT training, two sets with progressively increasing resistance. On Tuesday and Thursday, do one hour of recreational sport or aerobics. On Saturday (or Sunday), enjoy several hours of more vigorous outdoor activity with friends/family.

- Daily healthy eating as scheduled.
- Daily entries in your exercise, food, and thought journals.
- Same end-of-week routine, with added attention to your thought journals to monitor for depressed mood, out-of-norm anxiety, or repeated self-sabotage.

Dr. Huizenga Recap—Week Nine

You've Come a Long Way, Baby!

The 36 State Home Team has proved an important point. It's no cakewalk, but you can lose substantial amounts of fat at home, eating regular store-bought food and continuing your normal, busy lives. At this point, amazingly, the home team is on track to nearly equal the fat loss of the televised contestants on *The Biggest Loser-1*! And you're doing it on your own—staying consistent with your calorie allotments and post-

---

Week-Nine Totals for the 36 State Home Contestants:

Average Week-Nine weight loss: women, 4 pounds (1.9%); men, 5 pounds (1.6%)

Average total weight loss: women, 30 pounds (12.3%); men, 50 pounds (14.8%)

---

exercise anabolic shake, without trainers putting you through your paces, with less exercise per day, fewer injuries, and less emotional duress than the contestants at the ranch!

Translation? You've come a long way, baby! You've reached the equivalent of half a "stomach weight-loss surgery." You've already lost about one-third of your excess fat. Your fat loss is right on target, but you still have a long way to go to reach your WOW! weight. This is no time to

Table 9.2 Women's Individual 36 Home Team
Member Statistics

Women's Starting Weights	Weight At 2 Months	Weight-Loss Percentage
286.4	259.0	9.6
276.6	230.0	16.8
270.3	251.0	7.1
269.7	221.5	17.9
267.8	238.0	11.1
263.3	256.0	2.8
255.5	233.0	8.8
252.1	226.0	10.4
246.9	223.0	9.7
246.3	222.0	9.9
241.8	204.0	15.6
240.8	204.5	15.1
234.3	202.0	13.8
232.5	207.0	11.0
231.7	189.0	18.4
227.4	174.0	23.5
221.4	199.0	10.1
213.9	182.0	14.9
213.8	199.0	6.9
210.9	189.4	10.2
195.8	174.0	11.1
Women—Total Averages		
242.8	213.5	12.1

Table 9.3 Men's Individual 36 Home Team
Member Statistics

Men's Starting Weights	Weight At 2 Months	Weight-Loss Percentage
410.3	340.0	17.1
402.7	365.0	9.4
398.0	334.0	16.1
367.0	339.5	7.5
366.1	285.0	22.2
355.7	298.0	16.2
353.1	301.0	14.8
326.0	293.0	10.1
325.3	281.0	13.6
323.4	247.0	23.6
306.5	273.0	10.9
298.1	241.0	19.2
293.7	241.5	17.8
292.4	265.0	9.4
268.0	216.0	19.4
Men—Total Averages		
339.1	288.0	15.1

apply the brakes! My goal is for each one of you to achieve your ideal body-fat percentage, essentially down to 40 pounds of fat for women and men (the smaller women will still have more fat per total weight because women are "ideal" at about 25 percent, men at 15 percent body fat), at the end of our health crusade.

The next two-month stretch won't be easy, but, believe it or not, it will be easier than the first two months because:

- Your muscles have adapted to burn fat more efficiently.
- You are now physically fit and athletic enough for more vigorous exercise.
- You are now mentally fit. You have more confidence and are less hesitant to apply coping skills.
- You've got a strong foothold in nutrition, having learned important

shopping secrets, how to prepare food in advance, and how to count calories.

- You've established regular workout routines, better eating and sleeping regimens, and, surprisingly, your families and coworkers are (mostly) not only supporting you, they're inspired and impressed by your dedication. Of course, unfortunately, there are also people lurking in the peripheries of your lives who are jealous—literally licking their lips just waiting for you to slip up.

Week Nine Adjustments

As you begin Week-Nine, make the following adjustments:

P.M. Exercise: Increase Your PPT Training

We're now going to double both the time and attention spent on strengthening and shaping with the PPT training. The plan is to increase from the current 30 minutes on Monday, Wednesday, and Friday to 50 minutes (after a 10-minute aerobic warm-up), with a renewed emphasis on progressively increasing the resistance. Obviously, muscle retention hurts absolute weight loss, so if your only goal was to win a weight-loss contest, you'd never touch a barbell. But you're doing this for optimal fat loss, health, cosmetics, and mainly fat maintenance. Right?

Stay On Your Current Calorie Allotment

True, the women have already lost 30 pounds, on average, the men 50, and you're aware that diet experts and diet books claim that you now should proportionally decrease your calorie intake. Wrong! Not with The WOW! ℞. Since lean tissue burns essentially all the calories (fat only burns a tiny fraction) and since this new approach to weight loss preserves lean tissue, for the first time when large amounts of weight are lost, "dieters" don't need to cut their caloric allotment because not only has lean tissue been maintained—in most instances muscle has been gained!

Enter a Three-Day Food Journal Into a Food Journaling Internet Site or Reconsult a Dietitian (RD)

At this stage of the program, it's important to make sure you're getting enough protein (one gram per pound of lean tissue), enough variation in your fruits and vegetables, and enough micronutrients, such as calcium, iron, and antioxidants. Also, consult a dietitian if you still don't have the confidence to properly calculate calories while eating in a restaurant.

Perform a Mood Check

If you've lost less than 8 percent of your weight (women) or 10 percent (men) or you now recognize that you've been depressed all along, you should consult a psychologist. Exercise can be an effective treatment for some depression, but it may not be able to eradicate deeper disorders that can repeatedly derail meaningful weight-loss attempts. Someone once told me that he couldn't afford a psychologist; please remember, serious depression affects people in many ways—including earning money. Throw everything you can at depression—don't keep your head in the sand—numerous studies have shown that there is a major connection between obesity and mood disorders.

THE WOW! ℞—WEEK TEN

Follow Week-Nine Agenda with adjustments

Dr. Huizenga Recap—Week Ten

Wake Up, America: Our Physical Capabilities Are Huge!

As many as 20 million American TV viewers and millions more in 60 foreign countries have tuned in to *The Biggest Loser* and witnessed eye-popping body transformations. During Season Two, participants—with four-hour-a-day exercise and moderate caloric restriction—were "cured" of a veritable plethora of diseases by getting down to their WOW! weights

(35 percent weight loss over eight months). Amazingly, over 95 percent of the weight lost was fat (fat accounts for only 50 to 75 percent of weight loss on other diets and after bypass surgery). Despite these very visible, better-than-stomach-bypass accomplishments, obesity experts universally panned the TV show. They claimed gross overtraining ("What they're doing in this show is. . . working them at a pace they cannot sustain. . . I'd stake my life on this: Whatever weight these people lose, they'll gain right back"). They decried the "Pollyanna" weight-loss environment, which, because of the substantial cost of a live-in boot camp and the possible coercive nature of prize money, might not be easily applicable to the average overweight American. ("We can all agree our patients would be more successful at losing weight if they all had. . . personal trainers and access to well-equipped gyms whenever they wanted, and accountability in knowing that they were being filmed for national television. . . but is this reality or just a fantasy weight-loss experience?")

You can see why I was beyond curious about what would happen with our 36 home state folks who had none of the purported "overtraining" or "Pollyanna" weight-loss environment! Was four hours a day of exercise necessary for dramatic fat loss, or would two to two-and-a-half hours a day suffice? What are the overuse injury rates of each exercise approach? How much of the participants' dramatic fat loss can be attributed to the live-in weight-loss boot camp, the ever-present trainers or the prize money? And last but not least, would the contestants quickly put weight back on as the weight-loss experts had so emphatically "staked their lives (and reputations) on"?

Results! Drum roll, please. . .

The first-day medical exam observations of all 62 aspiring *Biggest Loser-3* contestants revealed the following:

- The BMI did not predict body-fat levels in this group. It's time doctors enter the 21st century and assess fat by determining accurate body-fat levels.
- The participants were sick: 79 percent were hypertensive, 6 per-

cent were diabetic, 24 percent were pre-diabetic, 29 percent were hypercholesterolemic, 18 percent were hypertrigyceridemic, and 11 percent smoked cigarettes. The real shocker? Despite pre-show clearances from their personal physicians, only 10 percent had ever been told they were hypertensive, 8 percent that they were diabetic or pre-diabetic, and 8 percent that they had elevated cholesterol levels.

- Metabolic syndrome, a particularly nasty predictor of early medical problems—when high blood pressure, diabetes, and high triglycerides occur simultaneously with an extra-large waist circumference—was seen in an eye-popping 62 percent of the participants. Curiously, this problem didn't necessarily occur in the fattest participants—it occurred in those with the highest percent of excess weight around the waist. So identifying regional fat patterns may be as important as identifying excess fat.
- Twenty-three percent of participants had been prescribed bariatric surgery. The surprise here? These 23 percent were significantly heavier, with higher BMIs, but not significantly fatter or sicker than the other participants who hadn't been considering stomach bypass or stapling surgery. None of these 23 percent had state-of-the-art body-fat determinations done. The moral? This isn't the first time patients and their doctors have been fooled by numbers, and it won't be the last. Again, never rely solely on simple weight or BMI to assess your need for bariatric surgery.

Week-Ten observations revealed:

- Weight-loss results of the boot-camp contestants and the home contestants dramatically exceeded those of the alternates, who were sent home without any instructions. Table 9.4 details exercise expenditures and caloric intakes of the boot camp, home, and alternate contestants.

Table 9.4 Exercise and Caloric Averages

	Women			Men		
	Boot Camp	**Home**	**Alternates**	**Boot Camp**	**Home**	**Alternates**
EXERCISE						
Total Daily[1]	3.8	2.3	0.8	6.0	2.3	0.2
Vigorous[2]	1.4	1.0	0.1	2.8	1.3	0
Moderate[3]	1.5	1.0	0.3	0.8	0.9	0.1
Walking	0.9	0.3	0.4	2.4	0.5	0.1
DIET						
Calories In	1,111	1,088		1,446.0	1,604	
% RDEE consumed[4]	69	70		62	70	

[1] *Total Daily Exercise:* the number of self-reported exercise hours performed six days per week.
[2] *Vigorous Exercise:* self-reported exercise intensity of jogging or greater (most listed weightlifting here).
[3] *Moderate Exercise:* self-reported exercise intensity less than jogging intensity (other than walking).
[4] % RDEE (Resting Daily Energy Expenditure) consumed: the number of calories consumed based on diet journals, divided by the calculated resting daily energy expenditure.

- Boot-camp women and men lost dramatic amounts of weight, consistent with prior seasons.
- The alternate men and women, on average, lost no weight, despite two women alternates actively participating in weight-loss programs (Meridia, Weight Watchers).
- Home participants—who, compared to their live-in boot-camp peers, had comparable caloric intakes but exercised and walked significantly less—lost nearly as much weight as their boot-camp peers! (Total weight loss trended 15 percent higher in the boot-camp participants, compared to home participants.) So the three-day weight-loss seminar, followed by a self-monitored home program consisting of intense exercise, strict adherence to individual-specific caloric guidelines, and post-workout shakes, were as predictive of dramatic fat loss as the prohibitively expensive live-in boot camp with 24/7 trainers, TV cameras, and financial incentives!
- Total weight loss of home participants who journaled faithfully was significantly greater than those who did not journal. (See Table 9.5.)
- Psychological surveys showed that the boot camp had a dark side: Isolation from family and work stressors proved to be counter-

Table 9.5 Total Weight-Loss Percentages—
Ten Weeks into *The Biggest Loser-3* Show

Sex	Boot Camp	Home Participants	Home "Nonjournalers"[1]	Home "Journalers"	Alternates
Female	15.2	12.3	10.2	14.6	0.7
Male	17.5	14.9	10.8	17.5	−1.5 (gain)

[1]Home "nonjournalers"—those with less than three weeks of completed calorie and exercise journals e-mailed in (10 of the 36).

productive, as participants edged toward depression without their families and home life.

- Boot camp and home participants—both with far less caffeine ingestion—got an equal boost in energy (which many called "boundless") compared with the alternates.
- Boot-camp participants each suffered, on average, two orthopedic injuries during the first two months—mainly knee, calf, ankle, and foot overuse ailments. The home-participant injury rate was fourfold less.
- Properly screened unfit obese and morbidly obese individuals were willing, and quite able, to quickly ramp up home exercise intensity and duration during the initial two months to a level consistent with 1 to 2 percent weekly weight loss, even with no ongoing supervision.
- Sedentary, morbidly obese individuals are capable of competitive, athlete levels of exercise. When they're motivated, they continue to exercise through transient overuse injuries. Based on two-month weight-loss results averaging 12 to 15 percent in home participants, it's reasonable to encourage substantially more strenuous exercise than the surgeon general's meager recommendations!
- This aggressive, pedal-to-the-floor exercise approach not only jump-started weight loss, it resulted in muscle gain in most instances—a huge plus. Muscle burns substantially more calories than fat, both during activity and at rest; therefore, weight-loss approaches that focus on maximum fat loss—with muscle gain—better position individuals for fat maintenance.
- Although many weight-loss doctors coach patients to set their weight-loss goals "realistically" low (i.e., at 5 to 8 percent, the upper end of percent weight loss seen in university-based, medically supervised weight-loss plans), safely getting participants as close to normal fat levels in as short a period of time as possible may

---

Week-Ten Totals for the 36 State Home Contestants:

Average Week-Ten weight loss: women, 2 pounds (1.0%); men, 4 pounds (1.3%)

Average total weight loss: women, 32 pounds (13.2%); men, 54 pounds (15.9%)

---

be advantageous; it may inspire people to maintain fat loss because they've had a life-changing health and cosmetic event.

- Despite repeated media pronouncements from experts guaranteeing that *Biggest Loser* participants and others who lose dramatic amounts of weight will quickly gain all their weight back, preliminary evidence—the one- and two-year follow-ups—suggest the opposite is true. Over the first year, contestants from the first three seasons on average kept off approximately 80 percent of all the weight they'd lost. The obesity "experts" appear to be basing their dire predictions on prior studies in which a big chunk of the weight lost was lean (muscle) tissue.

Wake up, America—we haven't scratched the surface of the physical capabilities of our overweight, obese, and morbidly obese citizens!

THE WOW! ℞—WEEK ELEVEN

Follow the Week-Nine Agenda with adjustments

Dr. Huizenga Recap—Week Eleven

Body Pain While Exercising, Questions and Answers

Question: During the past week, twice while I was running the third mile at an 11- to 12-minute pace, I started getting sharp pains under my right rib—not so bad that I would have to stop running altogether, but I am slowing down and it's messing up my pace. I've never experienced anything like this. Am I drinking too much water?

Answer: This sounds like a bowel or stomach stitch. When blood is diverted away from your bowel to muscles, the intestines sometime complain. It's not serious, but sometimes you need to slow all the way down to a walk until the cramp passes. Just to be totally safe, always check to make sure you don't have black stool (a sign of bowel bleeding). If the cramps recur, you may find your system requires you to fast (not eat) for up to four hours before strenuous exercise (some can tolerate calories in the stomach during exercise, others can't).

Although it happens rarely, cramps can result from hyponatremia—a potentially life-threatening water-salt imbalance—when an athlete loses salty sweat for hours on end (sweat can be instantly absorbed off your skin, so you don't always know how much you're sweating), even when he or she is drinking copious amounts of water. Again, when you lose lots of salt in sweat, and/or take in no salt with food and drink huge amounts of water, the body's sodium level may go haywire.

To be honest, I've seen drops in salt levels in about one-fourth of the contestants on *The Biggest Loser* ranch (rarely associated with cramps), who mistakenly believe they're doing the "right thing" by gulping down liters of water and then avoiding salt. Salt, by the way, does not add fat weight! Au contraire, proper salt and water levels are crucial for optimal fat burning!

Question: I'm having a hard time keeping my shoulders relaxed and I notice some tension in my neck and upper back when I've finished my runs. Occasionally, my right arm tends to feel as if it's numb, and my fingers start to tingle a bit. Usually I can shake it out, but it feels funny. Is this normal runner stuff?

Week-ElevenTotals for the 36 State Home Contestants:

Average Week-Eleven weight loss: women, 3 pounds (1.3%); men, 4 pounds (1.3%)

Average total weight loss: women, 35 pounds (14.3%); men, 58 pounds (17.0%)

Answer: Running is not something you automatically know how to do; it takes time (and sometimes coaching) to figure out how to "relax" while you're intensely working out. Try to stride gracefully, with fluid arm movements (it's a linear dance). If you feel yourself lean or hunch forward, clinch fists or become robotic, slow down and regroup. The silver lining is that when you run improperly (given the same speed and distance), you burn more calories due to inefficient body mechanics. The negative is that you can't go as far or as intensely for as long, the activity tends to be less enjoyable, and you're more at risk for injuries.

Your arm numbness probably represents low-grade nerve irritation at the level of the neck, elbow, or wrist. Emphasize good posture, and run with your shoulders back, chest forward, and arms open at your sides. You've explained that your arm numbness gets better during exercise and sometimes hurts when you are completely at rest, which indicates it's not heart related. Still, left-arm pain—or left-shoulder, upper-back, or jaw pressure that appears with exertion and disappears at rest—may signal angina, an acute insufficiency of blood to the heart muscle that can be a precursor of a heart attack and sudden death. Obviously, as an overweight person you are at increased risk of heart problems, although I've seen thin, optimally fit, world-class athletes get exertional angina, too. Yes, statistically, fit athletes are far less likely to have heart disease—but no one is completely immune.

If the tips I've offered don't promptly resolve the problem, or if you continue to experience upper body pain, consult with your physician.

THE WOW! ℞—WEEK TWELVE

Follow the Week-Nine Agenda with adjustments.

E-mails from the Heartland to Dr. Huizenga

"Yeah, I'm losing weight!" I umpire a lot of baseball. My uniform is now way too big, but since I'm not through losing weight, I haven't bought another one yet. Well, I was umpiring Saturday and I had to run from behind first base all the way over to third. On my way, my pants fell down! It was so embarrassing, but I was actually proud! I wanted to yell to everybody, "Yeah, I'm losing weight!" But I didn't. I just called the kid out and finished the game.

———— ————

Thinking about my two girlfriends that had the gastric bypass surgery, and all of the complications and drama that they have had to go through, makes me so glad that I didn't have the surgery. I have more energy and look more fit than they do. And I'm proud I'm doing it the old-school way—busting my butt—not surgically altering body parts, or other drastic measures.

———— ————

In reference to my involvement with the Body for Life program two years ago, I lost 16.5 total pounds in 12 weeks; I got suckered in on this one (other programs I tried, I either got bored or saw no quick results) and saw it to the end. I bought the Body for Life journal, the cookbook, videotape, etc., and the cases of the EAS protein drink mix

---

Week Twelve Totals for the 36 State Home Contestants:

Average Week-Twelve weight loss: women, 2 pounds (0.9%); men, 2 pounds (0.8%)

Average total weight loss: women, 37 pounds (15.1%); men, 60 pounds (17.7%)

(lots of $$$). I have to admit, at the end of the 12-week program, I did not look like the inspiring book-jacket photos. I did not get the body they said I would, but I did not complain, I just figured I did something wrong, even though I followed their program to a "T."

Dr. H., there is no comparison to your program. With a valid starting point and short continual goals, along with proper nutrition and exercise, you and your staff have helped me lose, in 12 weeks, from 294 lbs to 234.5, a total weight loss of 59.5 pounds. And, I have to admit, your program is a lot more fun, and in the same time frame I have lost four times as much weight, with less time spent in the gym. Oh, I forgot to ask, do you sell cases of your anabolic shakes? (Just joking).

——— ——

For the first time in my life, I've overcome obstacles and am keeping the weight off. I'm excited about what I feel like and what I will look like—I will finally have my outside match the beauty inside me. The sense of accomplishment that I feel is indescribable. Before, I would never have dreamed that I could accomplish any of this. It's a good feeling.

——— ——

A major high came at the end of last week. I completed my second triathlon. I finished in 1:32:59, which was almost a 10-minute improvement from the first one, one month ago! I'm amazed that I am feeling as well as I do, considering the pounding my body is taking. I have no physical ailments at this time. One thing that is awesome, that I recently noticed, is that I have not had any allergy symptoms over the last six to eight weeks. I don't know what impact weight loss would have on allergies, but it's been great. When I look back at the week as a whole, I can still say that I have strictly kept to my calorie count and diet (with no lapses) and continue to come in under my allotted calories. . . with no hunger! I'm very pleased with the fact that we've added more weight training. Yes, I'm after those guns!

——— ——

Doc H., I'm going to continue to follow your plan (full calorie intake, two hours workout intense with half of an anabolic shake immediately after. . . as opposed to four hours exercise and less calories (as I had been doing) and see if I can continue to bump up my weight loss (I still don't understand how in the world I was able to lose more with less). I'm enjoying the new push-pull-twist workout and am beginning to see definition in my legs and arms (which is a miracle. . . I have never had defined arms in my life!). I am strutting my stuff, believe me.

——— ——

My weight this morning was 211. I am okay with that because I am now weighing in before I exercise in the morning. I always weighed in directly after the workout that allowed me to drop additional weight. Basically, it was like you were saying, water weight doesn't matter; I don't have to dehydrate trying to "fool" myself on my weekly weigh-in day anymore.

——— ——

I don't want to jinx anything, but it feels like things are on autopilot. Even over the holiday weekend, which my family and I spent at a friend's house on a lake, I gave them a heads-up on what I prefer to eat, and it was pretty easy to stick with. . . even passing on the alcohol was relatively simple. Of course, it helps that I am surrounding myself with only my best of friends and they are super supportive. I'm not going through shock anymore when I see my weight go down on the scale or when I put on my clothes. I guess I'm accepting that this is my way of life now and not some new fad I'm trying.

——— ——

My ex-wife told me the other day: "When your face was 'heavier,' it brought your cheeks in and almost gave you a frown when you were not talking or smiling. So it gave the appearance that you were always grumpy. But now that your face is thinning out, there is almost always a smile there. And it looks like you are so much more happy."

So maybe our bodies are showing the real people that were hidden away. . . no?

——— ——

I'm sure a lot of us are only halfway to our "goal" WOW! weight. Is it hard for any of you to field so many compliments now? I think at times our minds (at least mine) want to listen to the compliments and say, "You know, I do look better"—rather than focus on the ultimate goal that we have all set. Maybe I'm overreacting, but I'm really tired of people asking me if I feel better now that I've lost, or asking how much better I feel. On the one hand, I enjoy the compliments, but when they ask this I keep wondering, in the back of my mind, how they thought I felt before I started working out. Do they think I was miserable? 'Cause I was (and am) a pretty happy guy!

——— ——

This last weekend, I got in a kayak and was off and paddling like I had been doing this for quite some time. It was an awesome feeling gliding over the lake and knowing I had total control over how fast and which way I went in the kayak. What a great upper-body workout. Not only would I have never tried that when I was heavier, I probably couldn't have even begun to get into a kayak. Oh, actually, I might have gotten in, but I know it would have been almost impossible to get my fat butt out of it. The opening in a kayak is very small.

——— ——

Is it possible I could be feeling less hot? I know this sounds nuts, but I seriously feel less warm when I'm outside in the muggy heat than I used to. We're all exposed to this lovely, muggy weather seemingly drowning the country in sweat. . . is anyone else experiencing the same thing? I just feel like every time people are complaining about how unbearable it is, I'm not as uncomfortable as I remember being in the past.

This is making me curious. . . at the start of the show, how many of us picked out "goal" clothing items that weren't small enough? I fit in mine already, so I've decided on another one, but it's kinda weird to me. Apparently I just didn't believe in myself enough?

———— ————

Good news this morning. I put on my goal outfit and it fit! I haven't worn this dress for five years! The skirt is loose now! So, my new goal item is a size 10 leather skirt. . . that I wore when I was in college! Mind you, three months ago I couldn't zip the skirt around one of my thighs! So the long and short, or the fat and skinny, is. . . many miles traveled, yet still many miles to go to my WOW! weight!

———— ————

I had the same "problem" (a good problem to have!). I'm wearing my goal item to a wedding this weekend! I think it wasn't that we didn't believe in ourselves, but more that it's just hard to conceptualize the amount of weight we're losing! I don't even know the last time I weighed what I eventually want to weigh, so I had no idea how that would translate into a clothing size! I just took a guess and grabbed the smallest size I ever remember being!

———— ————

An epiphany of sorts about my life, where I've been and where I am heading: When I was seriously overweight and eating what I wanted, I basically numbed myself with the amount of food that I ate. Now, I am living life at face value and dealing with things that the roller coaster of life has to offer. Oddly enough, for the first time in my life, when I'm feeling stressed and anxious, I am not even hungry.

———— ————

My big race is Friday night. I wish, Doc H., you could run it with me—I'm pretty sure I'll need some sort of medical intervention—or at least someone to pick me up off the ground at the end! I did a practice run on Sunday and it took me 2 hours and 40 minutes. I thought I would die. I am hoping to do it in 2.5 hours. If it wasn't for all the support from this group and Doc H.'s words of encouragement, "fat people can do it, it just takes longer and hurts more!," I would never have thought this dream would become a reality. No more sitting on the sidelines eating doughboys and drinking beer.

——— ———

I ran a 10K this weekend in 1 hour 12 minutes. It was rather exciting, because the most I have ever run straight without stopping to walk for a minute was 3 miles. . . so to run 6.2 straight through with one 30-second water break was a big feat! Now I'm hooked!

——— ———

All right, I think I have a small victory to share, too! Tonight I have a running date! That's right, no movies, no dinner and drinks, we're going running! Never in 1,000 years would I have expected that to be my idea of a fantastic date! And here's the wildest part. . . he's worried about being able to keep up with me! (I'm sure he has nothing to worry about yet. . . I'm not doing any 10-minute miles yet!) But still, the idea that someone who didn't know me before actually sees me as somewhat athletic, or at least active, is wild! He's never seen me any other way, so he just assumes that's how I am!

——— ———

Guess who ran her first 10-minute mile? The fattie who was always last during the presidential physical fitness test. . . changing alone in the girls' locker room, while everyone else who'd finished miles ahead was already in class. . . think I'll go cry quietly in my anabolic shake now. . . (tears of joy, of course).

——— ———

So, this Saturday I get to see the love of my life. I haven't seen him in two years. So I decided that since it's a big occasion, I get to buy some new clothes! It was so exciting. I spent two solid hours trying on just about everything and didn't go home upset that I looked awful in everything I tried on. So I have a hot new outfit to wear for my boy.

And I'll definitely be rocking it at his concert. . . yes. . . the Justin Timberlake concert. I've got me a seat right next to the stage and I am so excited. Who needs to pay bills when you can spend $160 on an outfit and a ticket to see a hottie!

THE WOW! ℞—WEEK THIRTEEN (THE HALFWAY MARK!)

Continue the Week-Nine Agenda with the Following Halftime Adjustments:

1. At home, repeat your body composition data:
   - Weigh yourself first thing in the morning.
   - Measure your waist circumference (parallel to floor at level of belly button after a breath out).
   - Take whole-body bathing-suit pictures (two-piece for women) from the front, side, and back at exactly six feet away for refrigerator-door comparison.
   - Goal clothes: Can you fit into them yet? Did you underestimate your ability to lose fat? Is it time to pick new goal clothes?

2. Repeat your body-fat percentage measurement (preferably via iDEXA, DEXA, underwater weighing, or Bod Pod).

3. Calculate your current RDEE, minimum calorie allotment, and WOW! weight, and answer these questions:

   - Has your estimated resting daily energy expenditure (RDEE) changed?
   - Has your individualized daily minimum calorie allotment changed?
   - Has your estimated WOW! weight changed?

Week-Thirteen Totals for the 36 State Home Contestants:

Average Week-Thirteen weight loss: women, 2 pounds (1.1%); men, 3 pounds (1.1%)

Average total weight loss: women, 39 pounds (16.0%); men, 63 pounds (18.6%)

---

4. Reassess your thought journals for eating or mood disorder; consult with psychologist early, not late, in the process if you feel you have problems.

5. Exercise.

A.M. workout: Continue to ramp up intensity. (Great insight by your teammates who noted stalled progress when they got "too comfortable during exercise.") Add interval aerobics (speed work) for two to three of the morning sessions to amp up the "afterburn."

Following are walking exercises that equal 5 mph jogging intensity for those unable to run:

- 3 mph walk at 13 percent grade
- 3.4 mph walk at 10 percent grade
- 3.8 mph walk at 8 percent grade
- 3.8 mph walk at 6 percent grade, with ankle weights (1 pound for each 100 pounds of your weight)
- 4 mph walk at 7 percent grade
- 4.5 mph at 4 percent grade
- 3.8 mph level walk on sand or hard snow

PM workout:

- One hour PPT training three times a week—progressively increase the resistance.

- More aerobics two to three times a week or attempt to participate in a camaraderie sport such as tennis, volleyball, soccer,
group cycling, or hiking.
- Consider a two- to three-hour less-intense aerobics session/na-
ture encounter (preferably with family or friends) on Saturday
or Sunday. Golfing counts if you walk the course—extra credit
for carrying your clubs.
- Move during your workday! Stand up during meetings, pace during phone calls (or do some of your calf and hamstring static
stretches), walk to coworkers instead of using phones or e-mail.
- Move while doing household chores. Dance while you do the
dishes; move around while watching television instead of loung-
ing on the sofa; view yard work as a workout, not a chore, etc.
All of this may sound silly, but some of our most successful
weight losers have fidgeted and moved nonstop to the point of
being accused by friends and coworkers of being hyperactive.

Dr. Huizenga Recap—Week Thirteen, The Halfway Mark

What Are Your Real Goals? Are You Willing to Stay the Course for a
Few More Laps?
You've battled through a summer of blistering heat to continue your
quest to look great, feel younger, and live longer. Halfway through our
body-transformation marathon, the women have lost a sizzling 16.0 percent, the men a scorching 18.6 percent of their original body weight. Excellent! No wonder many of your goal clothes already fit. But from day
one I said we were striving for more. The goal is your WOW! weight. For
our group, that translates to a 30 to 35 percent weight loss—less if you
manage to add muscle in the face of fat loss; possibly more if you under-
cut your calorie allotment or overexercise and cannibalize muscle for fuel.

As expected, we've had a few teammates stumble here and there,
but let's face it, maintaining a rigid exercise and healthy eating plan

is (literally) no walk in the park! Screw-ups will happen, but to be successful you must develop and use your coping strategies to quickly recognize self-sabotage and right the ship.

Question-and-Answer Time

Question: How accurate are the calorie-counting tools on a treadmill? I usually input my weight, age, etc., so that I can see how many calories I'm burning. When I did hill intervals at 3.8 mph at a 0-to-10-percent incline for 1.5 hours, it said I burned 750 calories. It seemed like a lot, so I wasn't sure if it was accurate. Does this sound about right? If so, if I'm eating 1,100 calories a day, is it okay to burn 750 or more a day—on a regular basis? Thanks!

Answer: I know your weight is now down around 175, so I did a little research. If the "average" incline was about 4 percent over the 90

Table 9.6 Gross Calories Burned per Hour
(includes basal calories)

Your Weight	Rest	Slow Walk	Walk	Brisk Walk	Jogging
	Watch TV	3 mph	3.5 mph/4 mph	4.5 mph	5 mph/6 mph
150	68	225	259/340	429	544/736
175	79	262	302/397	500	635/858
200	91	299	345/454	572	726/981
225	102	337	388/510	643	816/1103
250	113	374	431/567	714	907/1226
275	125	412	474/624	786	998/1348
300	136	449	517/680	857	1,089/1471
350	159	524	603/794	1000	1,270/1716
400	181	599	689/907	1143	1,451/1961

minutes and you didn't hold onto the rails, ever, that number is only about 10 percent inflated, but close enough. Unfortunately, the digital displays on exercise equipment are just as often wrong as right.

Actually, getting an accurate caloric burn rate for something as simple as walking on a flat, firm surface is tough. I Googled "calories burned per hour" and typed in a "one-hour walk at 4 mph for a 200-pound woman," and got nine different answers on the first ten sites: 454, 408, 345, 432, 764 (from the site of St. Johns Medical Center, Longview, Washington), 325 (only a 150-pound woman was listed), 345, 215, 529 (Web MD), 208 (fitday.com)—ouch! My exercise physiology textbook left a little to be desired, too. It gives three separate readings: 420, about 420, and 528. You get the picture. Exercise calorie counts are not yet an exact science.

Believe it or not, exact numbers for walking speeds from 3 to 4.5 mph and the values for people over 200 pounds are still a little in doubt; even under the best of circumstances, there's a 15-percent error rate. Secondly, there are huge individual variations based on your skill, stride length, height, age (child, adolescent, or adult), pace, fitness level, hydration, and nutritional status. And have you ever seen a treadmill that accounts for the diminished calorie burn from the mechanical advantage of the spinning belt or rail handholding?

Lastly, there's always confusion about whether the number given is gross (all the calories burned during the hour of exercise) or net (the extra calories burned over and above what you'd use sitting on the couch watching TV). Table 9.6 gives some gross-calories-burned guidelines.

The second part of your question is also tricky. Before observations of *The Biggest Loser* participants, before watching some of them regularly exercise off over 3,000 calories on 1,500- to 1,800-calorie diets, no one had an answer. Amazingly, it turns out that it's fine to burn 750 calories or more during your exercise sessions when consuming only 1,100 calories daily—if your healthy eating plan has primed your system to burn off the 750 calories as fat, not muscle. Protecting muscle includes a slow ramp-up of weightlifting, prompt replenishment of energy stores, and critical body-building blocks via the protein-carbohydrate anabolic shake immediately after each exercise session and proper nutrition during the remainder of the day, too.

Remember, if you're starved, carbohydrate deficient, or dehydrated, you put yourself at risk for medical side effects—and you aren't optimizing your fat-burning system.

Question: Contrary to others in the group, I'm not doing so well. The scale is not moving! I've been at the same weight for three weeks now. I'm extremely frustrated and upset by this. On many days I go under my calorie limit (eat closer to 900 calories). Two times—two weeks ago—I messed up and had two vegan-everything-oatmeal-all-natural cookies. I tried to balance it out by exercising for one more hour and not eating anything else for the rest of the day. Otherwise, I stick to the program every day! Typically I do not drink an entire shake, and sometimes I skip dinner if I am working out. Anyhow, I was wondering if you could look at it and tell me how to improve. I really wanted to lose more weight during July. Help. . . please!

Signed, Stuck on Flat Terrain in the Midwest!

Answer: You have a typical (but maddening, nonetheless) complaint: Your weight loss appears to have plateaued! This is when dieters cuss and swear that their metabolism has changed because they've been faithful to their diet and exercise. Sadly, sometimes at this crossroads, your friends, your spouse, and your doctor (who naively are trying to help, but their tactics are, more often than not, counterproductive) start wondering if there's a little cheating going on behind the scenes. True, there may be "hibernation" phenomena in diet-only weight-loss programs, whereby your body responds by becoming substantially more fuel efficient, but you can combat this with vigorous exercise.

Table 9.7 Stuck on Flat Terrain for the Last Three Weeks

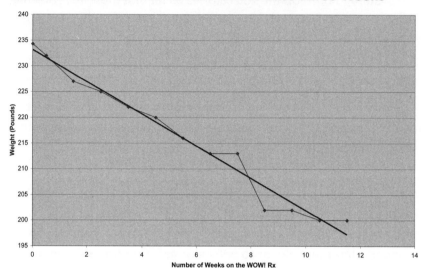

Number of Weeks on the WOW! Rx

However, I sense there's a less-sinister explanation. One possibility: You are obviously undereating and mis-timing your nutritional intake. Two, please look at your weight-loss graph, Table 9.7:

Part of the answer to your current "pseudo plateau" begins with what was clearly an inappropriately large weight loss around the eight-week mark. Remember, I talked to you shortly after that big weight-loss week, when you were feeling spent/lethargic/too punk to exercise. You were clearly calorie-and-glycogen (carbohydrate) depleted, given your increased exercise. Additionally, you weren't optimally timing what calories you did take in, i.e., you drank no anabolic shakes after you exercised. Subsequently, after an off-exercise day and two days of in-creased calories (refilling your glycogen fuel tanks while also increas-ing your weight with this "heavy" but vital fuel), you felt great, raring to go at exercise and all of life.

Three, look at the math. When you had the big weight-loss week, around five of those pounds were simply water released with the glycogen. Per my request, you loaded back up on glycogen and gained around five pounds of water; however, your weight stayed the same

228

for those several weeks, meaning you lost around five pounds of fat to equal the water you were appropriately restoring. Draw a "best" straight line through your weight loss. You're only a few pounds heavier than expected based on your body's established metabolism!

Moral of the story? Sometimes a "really big" weight-loss week is not all it's cracked up to be. Over and over, I've seen patients who were blown away weeks later by the "inevitable water reload." It leads not only to the self-doubts you expressed, but actually convinces the dieter to throw in the towel, saying, "I quit! This program does not work! I'm doing everything right and I didn't lose a single pound!" But now you know all about how you can be fooled by your scale weights (ups and downs) and the fact that exercise combats your body's "hibernation" response to weight loss.

Stay the course. Stop the "I'll never shed another pound" worrying. Ten bucks says you'll break through in the next one to two weeks.

THE WOW! ℞—WEEK FOURTEEN

Stay with the Halftime Agenda

Dr. Huizenga Recap—Week Fourteen

First off, congratulations are in order for Mr. Triple Digits—our first 100-pound loser. His waist, 56 inches at the onset, is now sporting 40-inch pants, although he tells me he's still got gut protruding above the belt line and a way yet to go to his WOW! weight.

Secondly... drum roll, please. STUCK ON FLAT TERRAIN IN THE MIDWEST! had a breakthrough week!

"The scale finally moved—3 pounds since Sunday! Dr. H., I cannot tell you how much your help has meant to me these past few days. I was

---

Week-Fourteen Totals for the 36 State Home Contestants:

Average Week-Fourteen weight loss: women, 2 pounds (1.0%); men, 3 pounds (0.9%)

Average total weight loss: women, 41 pounds (16.9%); men, 66 pounds (19.4%)

---

really frustrated, and you gave me hope. I am more determined than ever to reach at least a 30-percent weight loss and I'd like closer to 40 percent! I just have to figure out how to do it without overdoing it. I guess it's called perfection. Well, many miles to go. . . Again, thanks so much!"

Questions and Answers

Question: I'm still overweight, but now I feel great! Should I be taking vitamins? Do you take them?

Answer: Want to see your doctor dance? Then ask, "What vitamins should I take?"

In the 1980s, when I opened a practice, it was easy. "I don't know," I'd say. "Your best bet is fresh fruit, vegetables, whole grains, and lean protein, including three fish meals per week and nonfat milk products—even if you're on a low-calorie diet. You don't want to depend on vitamins. They don't have all the good things from food—heck, we don't know what all the good things are in food. Even if we did, we'd still be clueless about nature's proprietary blends—the exact ratios of vitamins, antioxidants, phytonutrients, and minerals that have repeatedly been shown to prevent cancer, heart disease, and hypertension in studies comparing high to low fruit and vegetable intake."

Then things got confusing—like when the Pope declared that eating meat on Friday was no longer a sin. Overnight, a discovery of a modern-day deficiency turned the vitamin field, and doctor's recommendations, upside down.

First, a 1991 study proved that having moms-to-be take a daily folic acid supplement could drastically reduce a rare neural birth defect. Okay, the folic acid would help just 2,000 of the 1,000,000 babies born in the United States each year, but this revelation was still a shocker. A vitamin deficiency disease in modern America. . . with ample folic acid supplied by green leafy vegetables, lentils, and beans?

We've all read about beriberi in alcoholics, scurvy in sailors, and rickets in impoverished children, but that was in the dark ages of vitamin knowledge, the prehistoric 1800s, before we knew about vitamins B, C, and D. The last deficiency disease in America, seen in parts of the south in the 1930s, was corn- and rice-diet induced pellagra, which was eradicated by state-mandated B_3 (niacin) enrichment of flour.

One more shocker came in 1991. Excess homocysteine, a breakdown product of protein, was shown to increase the risk of cholesterol-clogged arteries three- to fourfold, and folic acid and other B vitamins were the keys to detoxifying homocysteine. Other studies followed confirming the vital role of B vitamins. More heart disease and cancer were seen when levels of dietary folic acid, and to a lesser degree B_6 and B_{12}, were low.

Bottom line, you can get the needed 0.4 mg of folic acid in a balanced diet, but most Americans take in only 0.2 mg in vegetables, plus an extra 0.1 mg from grains since the U.S. government began a 1998 food fortification program. No one is sure whether the current average American intake of 0.3 mg is enough.

But it was the third scientific happening, the "free-radical theory of aging," that caused doctors to be starry-eyed over the unlimited potential of "antioxidant" vitamin supplements. Simply put, the free-radical theory casts oxidants as the ugly arch enemy. They damage our cells. They age our DNA. They can kill us. We can see oxidation when

iron rusts or a fresh-cut apple turns brown. We smell it as nonrefrig-
erated fish goes rancid. Oxidation is harder to detect in our bodies,
but rest assured, it is occurring everywhere, all the time. Our skin is
oxidized from sun and X-ray radiation, our lungs from cigarette smoke
and air pollution, our guts from ingested chemicals, our joints from
arthritis inflammation, and our entire systems from constant battles
with sugar spikes and infection.

Energy generation—the very core of our existence—is the number one
oxidant offender. Our cellular engines, the mitochondria, efficiently
combust fat, carbohydrate, or protein fuels with oxygen, but they're
not perfect. Like power plant smokestacks, they spew pollution, most
notably unstable oxygen molecules called free radicals. These toxic
by-products form by the thousands each second in every cell in our
bodies, and unless instantly neutralized, like irksome gnats, they bite
into surrounding tissue. If it's a blood vessel, free radicals might damage LDL—the "bad" cholesterol—and twist the molecule into stickier
glue that promotes vessel damage, setting a course toward blockage.
If it's DNA that's zapped, a series of naked nucleotide switches are
all that stand between a serene cell and an angry cancer.

The body, in its wisdom, devised a multitiered defense. One level of
protection involves hundreds of unique antioxidant vitamins tucked
with military precision into defensive positions around valuable cellular real estate. For millions of years, we've stolen antioxidant de-
fenders from fresh fruit, vegetables, and grains (plants can't survive
without armies of carotenoids, flavonoids, and vitamins C and E to
shield their vital cell structures from sunshine oxidants). When observational studies showed that the levels of antioxidants in our diets
predicted the chance of getting heart disease, cancer, and brain deterioration, a mad race was on to mega supplement for eternal health.

Sadly, human trials with large doses of beta-carotene and vitamins C
and E have shown no benefit over placebo—and could possibly cause

harm. There has been a lot of finger pointing in scientific circles, but no one knows exactly where we went wrong. The consensus is as follows: The free-radical theory of disease and aging is still valid, but nature has hundreds of specialists in its antioxidant armies, so it's not surprising that simplistic supplementation—high doses of one or several antioxidants in isolation—does not match the benefits of an abundant fruit and vegetable diet.

The following may be more information than you bargained for, but the vitamin E story is illustrative of the complexity of human systems and the naiveté of our band-aid treatments. Natural vitamin E is a delicate balance of eight isoforms, right-handed gamma in higher concentrations than right-handed alpha-tocopherol. To sum up, natural and synthetic forms of vitamin E are not the same, including the fact that there's no freshness guarantee with capsulated synthetic vitamin E, which can go rancid (oxidized)! But most of the vitamin E studies have been conducted using synthetic (not natural) vitamin E, with no freshness guarantee. Why? It's far cheaper. Natural vitamin E has no patent protection, so there's no profit incentive to do these studies correctly.

I'm pragmatic now when asked, "What vitamins should I take?" Some people, even in affluent Beverly Hills, don't follow optimally balanced, nutrient-complete diets. People who have less disposable cash may try to "eat healthy," but be unable to afford good-quality fresh fruit, vegetables, whole grains, and lean protein. Therefore, a multivitamin-multimineral with the U.S. recommended daily allowance (RDA) of vitamins is safe, inexpensive (10 cents a day) and helpful for a portion of the population. Don't forget, though, high doses can have side effects. Even folic-acid supplements—the single vitamin proven to be beneficial beyond a shadow of a doubt—are not equivalent to "food" folate and may be a double-edged sword! Recent studies suggest, in folks over 65 years old, that folic acid supplements over 0.4 mg/day may actually hasten memory decline and increase the risk of colon cancer.

If your long-term health is a concern, why not step past self-supplementation and eat healthy? Why not get the full spectrum of anti-aging nutrients?

What I Recommend

- Make sure you consume the following core foods every day: Rotating colors of vegetables (4 to 6 servings plus) and fruit (2 to 4 servings); healthy fats (1 to 2 servings) and lean protein, including nonfat milk products (2 to 3 servings), poultry, soy products, or fish (3 servings a week minimum—select low-mercury species).
- If you are unable to consume the previous "core" foods on a regular basis, take an insurance multivitamin-multimineral supplying RDA levels of vitamins.
- Dieters (as well as alcoholics and the elderly) with poor or decreased nutrient intake and absorption require a multivitamin-multimineral with calcium (500 mg, men; 1,000 mg, women) and vitamin D (400 international units [IU]).
- People getting limited sun exposure, especially those living north of the San Francisco–New York latitudinal line, may benefit from vitamin D supplementation, especially if they are not getting adequate dairy and fish products.
- Avoid high-dose vitamin E—anything over 400 IU.
- No added iron for men or post-menopausal women.
- Vegetarians should consider iron, B_6, B_{12}, and calcium/vitamin D supplements.
- Menstruating women should consider supplemental iron.
- Moms-to-be or soon-to-be-moms-to-be should supplement 0.8 mg folic acid—but remember: This fat-loss program

is not safe or healthy for pregnant women and their babies! No one else should supplement with more than 0.4 mg/day.

- If you are diagnosed with age-related macular degeneration, specially formulated multivitamin-multimineral cocktails may slow the progression of your disease (however, taking the cocktail earlier has not been shown to prevent macular degeneration).

What You Should Do; What I Do

You are in the middle of a "diet," so you should take a multivitamin-multimineral with calcium and vitamin D.

I don't take supplements. Bottom line, I trust millions of years of evolution (food-born "complete" vitamins found in quality food) over today's vitamin manufacturers, some of whom sell synthetic products (i.e., vitamin E) with no assurance of comparability to naturally derived vitamins and no assurance of freshness.

That'll teach you not to ask me any more loaded questions, right?

THE WOW! ℞—WEEK FIFTEEN

Stay with the Halftime Agenda

Why Do Women Lose Proportionally Less Weight Than Men?
Women don't lose as much weight as men, even with equal effort. In *The Biggest Loser-1, 2*, and the *Special Edition* seasons, the men lost 11, 15, and 27 percent more weight than matched females, even when percent weight loss was used to adjust for the women's smaller initial body sizes. You can see from this week's 36 home contestants' stat board that, to date, our men's weight-loss percentage is running 14 percent higher than the women's, so history is, indeed, repeating itself.

Week-Fifteen Totals for the 36 State Home Contestants:

Average Week-Fifteen weight loss: women, 2 pounds (0.9%); men, 2 pounds (0.8%)

Average total weight loss: women, 43 pounds (17.6%); men, 68 pounds (20.0%)

Weight-losing advantage of men over women to date: 14%

Why do women lose less? No firm explanation exists, but there are multiple theories. One, it may be hormonal. Fat is needed for successful child bearing and rearing, therefore, female hormones may somehow conspire to protect fat. Two, as fat melts away, some have hypothesized that women may hang on to more fluid. My *Biggest Loser* data, however, shows that, on a relative basis, women held onto slightly less water than men. This phenomenon of women losing less weight is most likely a consequence of women carrying proportionally less muscle than their male counterparts. In fact, in our 36 home contestants, similar to prior participants, the women's bodies started out with 50.8 percent lean tissue to the men's 57.4 percent. Remember, lean tissue burns almost 10 times as much fuel as fat. Regarding the math, 57.4 is 13 percent more than 50.8. So on a pound-for-pound basis, the men started with 13 percent more fuel-burning capacity! It's not shocking, therefore, that the men also, on a pound-for-pound basis, lost about 14 percent more weight than their female counterparts.

THE WOW! ℞—WEEK SIXTEEN

Stay with the Halftime Agenda

Dr. Huizenga Recap—Week Sixteen

The Secret Behind Boundless Energy
Amazingly, you're still putting up world-class numbers as we stride, healthier and happier, into the second half of our fat-loss marathon. As

predicted, your pace has slowed a tad after the initial 10 weeks of the WOW! ℞, but I'm proud to say the 36 State Home contestants have pushed through the feared plateau phase and are still on track to achieve their WOW! weight. As a group we're knocking through some incredible milestones. . . but some of you are still neglecting to send in your exercise and calorie journals, and if you look at the following stats, I think you'll agree that there's still a little room for improvement.

Preliminary trends show that when individuals in the top one-third were compared to the bottom one-third of weight-loss losers, the top one-third:

- Journal their diet and exercise more
- Exercise more
- Drink less alcohol
- Note a greater drop in their TV time
- Follow a more regular schedule
- Self-report a greater increase in energy
- Are not younger or more "athletic" (based on their age, initial treadmill results, or number of high school varsity sports completed)
- Report no advantage to weighing in once a day, as opposed to once a week; of note, repeatedly weighing in more than once a day is typically a sign of trouble!

Week-Sixteen Totals for the 36 State Home Contestants:

Average Week-Sixteen weight loss: women, 2 pounds (0.8%); men, 3 pounds (1.1%)

Average total weight loss: women, 44 pounds (18.3%); men, 71 pounds (20.9%)

Top one-third: women, 25.9%; men, 29.2%

Middle one-third: women, 17.1%; men, 20.9%

Lower one-third: women, 13.2%; men, 15.0%

THE WOW! ℞—WEEK SEVENTEEN

Stay with the Halftime Agenda

Dr. Huizenga Recap—Week Seventeen

The 36 State Home Women Poised to Break Record!

The 36 State Home women have pulled even with the weight loss recorded by *The Biggest Loser—Special Edition* squad, who had two entire weeks of focused attention on the ranch and then personal fitness trainers at home. Congratulations!

Stay consistent. Stay focused. Look at yourself in the mirror and recognize your new priorities. You are now beginning to see how getting down near your ideal body fat is changing your lives. The collateral effect on your spouses, children, parents, friends, and even your pets is equally amazing and, perhaps, as rewarding as your own personal health accomplishments.

E-mails with Embarrassing Admissions

I've always been mad at the airlines. I've always hated to fly because every time my knees are painfully crammed into the seat in front, which always makes me mad; 'cause although I'm tall, at 6'2," I'm not that tall. I've repeatedly complained, "Why aren't these seats constructed for normal height people?"

Last week I had to fly for business. Guess what? Now that I've lost this massive amount of weight, my height is the same, but with my rear end a mile smaller, now my knees have plenty of room. . . . Funny, I never really considered that possibility.

Week-Seventeen Totals for the 36 State Home Contestants:
Average Week-Seventeen weight loss: women, 1 pound (0.6%); men, 2 pounds (0.8%)
Average total weight loss: women, 45 pounds (18.7%); men, 73 pounds (21.5%)

Dr. H.'s Embarrassing Admission

I've always considered myself empathetic to the plight of the overweight; I've heard enough of your stories to know that all too often you are the brunt of mean-spirited jokes or suffer not-so-subtle discrimination at work.

Toward the end of one of the early morning initial casting physical exams of *The Biggest Loser* contestants at my office, one of the doctors from the other side of my office comes in to work and is irate to see a contestant sprawled on the floor, blocking access to our radiology facilities. I get this other doctor's e-mail of this "unacceptable offense" and immediately storm out, upset because I've given very specific instructions to the show runners to manage all the extra traffic so as not to inconvenience the other doctors or their patients. After raising my voice to a production assistant, I find out the contestant was just on the ground temporarily—turns out because of his massive abdomen, it was physically impossible for him to put his shoes back on and tie them from a chair; he could only do it while sitting on the ground!

Talk about foot-in-mouth disease!

THE WOW! ℞—WEEK EIGHTEEN

Stay with the Halftime Agenda

Dr. Huizenga Recap—Week Eighteen

Please Journal!

Your fat loss and eventual successful fat maintenance are directly proportional to your time commitment, prioritization, preparation, mood, ability to identify and overcome obstacles, and the medical validity of The WOW! ℞ itself. While it's obvious that you need to exercise and eat correctly to lose fat, the role of writing down all exercise and food is still somewhat controversial. However, seeing is believing—check out Table 9.8 regarding the merits of journaling. Curiously, the 36 State Home contestants have "self-selected" into three groups:

1. "Noncounters"—10 of you (represented by the squares on Table 9.8) have never sent me more than one or two weeks of calorie and exercise records.
2. "First-half counters"—14 of you (the diamonds) started off journaling like gang busters, but over the last four to 10 weeks have stopped sending in exercise and calorie journals.
3. "Counters"—12 of you (the triangles) never stopped journaling.

The difference between the groups that keep track of their calories and exercise (counters and first-half counters) versus those who don't is pretty remarkable. The 10 (of the 36) contestants participating at home who elected not to journal from the beginning still lost weight—a few lost a lot of weight—but the average weight loss was only 60 percent of what counters lost. An interesting flashback: I discovered earlier that *The Biggest Loser-1*, *The Biggest Loser-2*, and *The Biggest Loser-Special Edition* noncounter contestants lost only 60 percent as much weight as counters after they were kicked off the ranch and sent home to continue on their own. Still, I never knew for sure if counting helped or if it was merely a marker for compulsive overachievers who would stick like glue to my two-a-day exercise and nutrition plan, regardless. Now I think I know.

Many of the 14 state contestants who have stopped journaling over the past one to two months ("first-half-only counters") are compulsive overachievers—in fact, five of the six highest weight losers over the first

Table 9.8 The Merits of Journaling

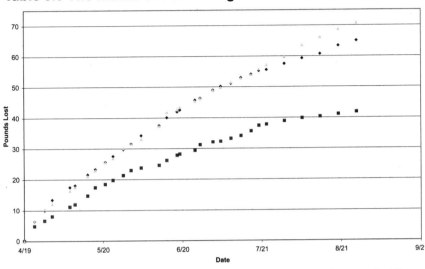

♦ 1st half counters (n=14) ■ Noncounters (n=10) ▲ 1st and 2nd half counters (n=12)

eight weeks have now flipped into the diamond clan. Have the folks in this group grown complacent about calorie counting? Are they thinking they no longer need to participate but can still lose fat? Has their mood or motivation changed? I don't know those answers, but clearly the data in Table 9.8 suggests that journaling helps to achieve the greatest fat-loss results, even among knowledgeable, motivated, overachieving, and regularly exercising participants.

In the last five weeks, while noncounters each lost about 5 pounds, the counters lost 15 pounds while the first-half counters—who had matched losses pound for pound with the televised ranch contestants through the first three months—faded off the pace, losing about 10 pounds. Interesting, huh?

The moral of the story? You really can help yourself! The fat you lose is proportional to your effort. You are in an enviable position; you have been given a road map to relatively quickly get down to your WOW! weight. Prioritize! Fill out your exercise, diet, and thought journals each week. Your life literally depends on it.

Questions and Answers

Question: I lost 2.5 pounds this week, but have a few questions. I have had no energy and my workouts have been suffering due to it. I go to bed hungry and wake up famished.

Answer: This has happened before to several of your teammates (most of the time with slowing of weight loss). You are not taking in enough calories and perhaps your percentage of carbohydrates consumed is too low as well, resulting in glycogen depletion. Take a full day off exercise; consume at least an extra hundred calories for lunch and dinner with special attention to getting in 50 percent of your calories as healthy carbohydrates (fruits, vegetables, and one to two whole-grain servings—a serving equals ½ cup), not the trashy, processed carbs. No one on this diet should be going to bed physically hungry—mentally hungry is another story. Ravenous in the morning is okay, but it means you need a little something (readily digestible) before your morning workout.

Question: A quick sex question. I've been told that running damages internal female reproductive organs and can affect fertility. Any truth to that?

Answer: Zero truth. Obesity lowers fertility and increases the risk of having a child with a birth defect. One of the neat things we've seen after the huge weight losses is that several contestants who've struggled beforehand to get pregnant have done so afterward.

Week-Eighteen Totals for the 36 State Home Contestants:

Average Week-Eighteen weight loss: women, 1 pound (0.6%); men, 4 pounds (1.4%)

Average total weight loss: women, 47 pounds (19.2%); men, 77 pounds (22.6%)

Sex issues associated with running include possible breast ligament stress and frequent testicular pain if respective proper support is not worn. One last sex-exercise tidbit: Exercise increases libido and certain strength regimens, specifically squats, enhance pelvic blood flow, and may have Viagra-like effects.

THE WOW! ℞—WEEK NINETEEN

Stay with the Halftime Agenda

Dr. Huizenga Recap—Week Nineteen

More E-mails from the Heartland

It's funny—people are asking me for diet advice and that is so weird! And I have already had a couple of clients tell me that I am their inspiration! Imagine if they really knew how hard I'm struggling. I have seen people out in public that I wish I could go up to and help. I have seen many guys who are in the same shape I was in. I want to be an inspiration and help many people. At my job I've worked the last 23 years making people pretty and feel better about their appearance, now it's time to help them feel better all the way to the inside. I want to be the Pied Piper!

——— ——

It was a shock the other day to see all of our before photos—with our shorts sucked up on our inner thighs. Man, I can't believe that we were all really that big! Anyhow, yesterday I was swimming with the kids while wearing a modest one piece with a skirt . . . (still not ready to show much skin) when a woman who was easily the size of my former self-plus . . . walked by me in a bikini. Yikes!

——— ——

Week-Nineteen Totals for the 36 State Home Contestants:

Average Week-Nineteen weight loss: women, 2 pounds (0.8%); men, 2 pounds (0.7%)

Average total weight loss: women, 48 pounds (19.9%); men, 78 pounds (23.1%)

I have started dating this guy and dating is a lot harder than I thought it would be (I have done very little dating in my 35 years). I have used my weight as a gigantic shield and don't really know what to do without it. Luckily, this guy is very understanding and is working on being more patient with me. He is very ready for marriage and children and I know that in my head I would like the same. However, I have never been so nervous, I don't feel ready for everyone. . . let alone the guy that I'm dating. . . to see who I was three months ago! Is anyone else feeling completely shy all of a sudden? I guess that I was at the lowest I could get before this weight-loss program. . . but now things are turning around and I'm not sure that I want everyone to see me the way I used to be. Anyone else feel a bit scared?

——— ——

Life is all about perception. How we choose to interpret things said to us is our choice.

I was a very competitive swimmer growing up and a coach once said to me, "Wow! You are really filling out." What I heard was, "Wow! Are you getting fat?" I actually told people that my coach called me fat for years, when in actuality it was my perception that he thought I was getting fat. . . and there started my eating disorder. I, too, fell into a rut. I became what I thought others thought of me.

Knowing when you're being a victim and deciding to change your outlook have been the most valuable lessons my mother has shared with me. I, too, am sharing it with my kids.

——— ——

I will always remember my grandma saying negative, nasty comments to me about my weight, always saying I was going to die from a heart attack before I was 10. I'd lie in bed as a child thinking I was having a heart attack—she had me convinced. The Xmas I turned seven, we went to her house as usual and I opened my gift, hoping for some cool, awesome gift. And when I opened the gift, she'd given me. . . a chintzy plastic gun and holster set that was obviously too small to fit me. My heart sank! I remember thinking: I wish I had a nice grandma.

Then like a scene out of an *Indiana Jones* movie, this large, brown belt whipped in front of my face. My mom had bought me this cool brown belt laced in silver, with this really cool buckle. She took the gun holsters and put them on the belt. Did I ever feel cool. I ran through that house like I was sheriff of Dodge City. I shot every outlaw in five states that day. There was a new sheriff in town!

I remember my "grandmonster" just glaring at me in disgust. She told me that if I kept getting fat I would have to get an even bigger belt. I have to say that if I truly ever hated anyone, she would be it.

My grandfather passed away and my mom literally abandoned that side of the family, so I didn't see my grandmother for about 25 years. Six years ago my mom called and told me she had passed away. When I went to the funeral home, I was so nervous about seeing this woman who had truly shaped my life. When I saw her in the casket, she was old and wrinkled and her hair was dyed jet black, just like I remembered it. Her eyes closed, she didn't have the glaring stare that once had intimidated me so bad. She was just a little, drawn-up, old woman. I guess I realized in her own way she just wanted me to be not only thin, but also healthy. I don't know if I'm just making excuses, but I really feel she knew what she wanted, but just didn't understand positive reinforcement, motivation, kindness, compassion, love. . . all of these would have worked so much better!

I made my amends that day, and threw hatred out the door. I walked out of there with a better understanding of myself. To this day my mom still has the brown belt and gun and holster set that took down many outlaws and robbers. . . and set me free! I tried putting it on a year ago and you know what? The old bitch was right—I was too fat for the belt! I should have known she would have had the last word.

But guess what? I weighed in today. . . I've lost almost all my fat! And as for every bank robber, outlaw, and all you damsels in distress, I'm finally getting healthy and fit. There really is a new sheriff in town!

——— ——

A few months ago, my doctor told me I should think about gastric bypass. I was so angry—at the time I was 30, and it just seemed way too drastic a step to take. However, the fact that he even was thinking about it with me has helped motivate me—to prove him wrong, to help wake me up to how serious my condition had gotten, etc. I do have to admit, though, the seeming ease of it all appealed to my lazy nature—have a surgery and magically lose the weight? Nice! But there's no such thing as a free, quick weight loss. . . I just read in the paper about some big study that showed weight-loss surgery costs $30,000 to $65,000 and that 40 percent of bypass surgery patients have a major complication within six months! I'm glad I turned down surgery. I like it this way. I pay the cost now and know exactly what it is: time, hard work, and sweat. I much prefer that to a sizable chance for some unknown complications later.

Dr. H., soon you will be able to put my before-and-after pictures up on your office wall with the heading, "Screw gastric-bypass, just keep moving!"

P.S. Please list me as "the funny one who shocked me with her dedication."

——— ——

Well, you all were talking about the input that you have been getting from people and the backhanded compliments. Well they strike again! One of my clients who I haven't seen in a while came today and said, "Oh my gosh you look great; you don't look a thing like yourself!"

—— ——

like when the facial expressions betray what people are saying. Their mouths are saying, "Wow! You look great," but their faces are saying, "Man! You were really fat!"

—— ——

I (obviously) still have belly flab (there was so much of it at the start that it will take ages, I think). Anyway. . . when my mom said, "I was telling your father that the style now seems to be for girls to have that belly flab hanging out, so you fit right in now! You look great!" (I know she meant well. . . but better phrasing maybe?)

—— ——

One of my family members recently said to me, "Wow! You are starting to look normal!" (Gee thanks, I think?)

—— ——

Part of me wonders if calling obesity an epidemic is the wrong choice of words. Does it convey the idea that it is a sickness? Are we taking away personal responsibility? If I get sick, it's because something else happened to me to cause it—I can't always help it. But weight is, for the vast majority of us, a result of overeating and a lack of exercise and understanding. If we take away the personal responsibility as a society, I think we will continue to see obesity rates growing faster and faster.

—— ——

I was on a small regional jet just before starting on this weight-loss plan. It is safe to say that they didn't have me in mind when they made this plane. Anyway, back to the story. The plane was sold out. It was a two-hour flight. Needless to say, my normal anxiety set in. Why?

The first thing is that I want to see if the seat belt is going to fit me. had to ask for an extension. I asked really low to the flight attendant "Can I have a seat belt extension?" Can you imagine what she did? Acting as though she didn't hear me, she blurted out loudly, "You need an extension!" I wished I was as small as I felt. As she gave me the seat belt extension, I hoped she could feel my utter disdain for her.

But you know, the more I think about it, I realize my anger was misdirected. I decided to get angry with myself. I decided I'd change.

THE WOW! ℞—WEEK TWENTY

Stay with the Halftime Agenda

Dr. Huizenga Recap—Week Twenty

The Weight-Loss Plateau. . . Is It What You're Eating or What's Eating You?

The 36 State Home Team had a little bit of an off week, losing on average 1.2 pounds, or 0.45 percent of your starting weight. The perplexing part is that nine individuals ($\frac{1}{4}$ of the entire group) chose not to send in their weights! (They were calculated in as a zero weight loss in the preceding calculations.)

Let's take a step back. Intense fat loss is a real chore. Sometimes it's just too much. The home team has already proven that sedentary obese individuals can achieve dramatic fat loss at home with an hour of exercise twice a day and moderate caloric restriction. Be aware, regardless of the reason you became obese—bad exercise and diet habits, bad genes, bad environment, situational stressors, mood (depression or anxiety) disorders, eating disorders such as binging or night noshing or all of the above—you're still miles ahead of your prior weight-loss attempts via low carbs, low fat, low "points," or very low-calorie liquid diets because:

- Your weight loss is now comprised entirely of fat—not muscle.
- Your habits are being reprogrammed! Never before have you been addicted to daily fat-loss exercise. Never before could you count calories or read labels. Never before did you grasp the rationale for intense exercise and what and when to eat.
- Regular exercise is an antidote for bad habits, bad genes, bad environment, life stressors, eating disorders, depression, or anxiety. Caloric restriction is not an antidote for any of the above, and eventually proves counterproductive. That's why no diet, no matter how well-intentioned or professionally structured, has ever been shown to result in long-term weight loss.
- People who lose large amounts of fat are more likely to keep it off than the usual dieters who initially lose on average a mere 2 to 5 percent of their weight with the currently popular home-based diets.
- Exercise is the only ticket to permanent fat loss—see the Week Twenty-Seven MAINTAIN! Plan on page 270.

Still, I can't bubble wrap your brains and shield you from each threat, or even the stretches of boredom, along the path to your optimal body-fat percentages (about 15 percent for guys, 25 percent for gals). But I do need to say this: All dieters struggle some of the time! Nobody is perfect! Believe me, dieters face a subconscious buzz saw of "get 'em-fat" brain signals tugging them back toward the adipose abyss. Curiously,

---

Week-Twenty Totals for the 36 State Home Contestants:

Average Week-Twenty weight loss: women, 2 pounds (0.8%); men, 1 pound (0.3%)

Average total weight loss: women, 50 pounds (20.6%); men, 79 pounds (23.4%)

---

some of these "get 'em-fat" neurotransmitters (melanocortin, neuropeptid Y, and others I can't spell), which help process metabolic satiety cues such as leptin and ghrelin, also modulate your mood and motivation! Who says eating and emotion aren't in cahoots?

Last week the e-mails from the Heartland struck a decidedly psychological tone. This week I talked to some of you and heard about:

- *Emotional eating.* Life keeps pitching curve balls, loved ones keep getting sick, marital crises, and over-the-top family picnics don't stop the minute you start The WOW! ℞. Sometimes even good stuff—like your "unexpected" fat-loss success—is hard to handle.
- *Depression.* Sometimes it's a down mood or too-easy tears and a glass-half-empty vision; sometimes it's subtler, with energy dips, inappropriate guilt, and sleep problems. If you're depressed, you have a twofold higher chance of becoming obese. If you're obese, you have a twofold higher chance of becoming depressed. If you're morbidly obese, there's a fourfold to eightfold increased chance of being depressed.
- *Body image alterations.* When you look at yourself and see something no one else sees, we could call this your "fat-person goggles." It takes months for your self-perception to adjust; stop looking in the mirror and evaluating every change in your body, your clothes, and your face. You are a work in progress!
- *Bingeing.* Loss of control, gaining and losing the same 10 pounds over and over.
- *Anxiety and frustration.* Being "out there" as a fat-loss role model to family and friends is an honor and a thrill, but it's also a real stressor. Stop already. . . for the umpteenth time, relax and smell the roses. . . enjoy your newfound energy!

But I don't want to put on airs. I'm no world-acclaimed psych authority.

Many of my insights are based on dealings with my patients'—and my own—mood swings, mostly with the help of an over-the-counter drug called *exercise*. (My psych training got off on the wrong foot because the month I was scheduled to do my fourth-year medical school Massachusetts Mental rotation, I had to fly out for a cross-country month of internship interviews. Okay, I made up an extra bunch of phony medical school interviews so I could spend the last two weeks in Haiti, San Juan, and St. Martin with my girlfriend—remember the unlimited 30-day plane tickets way back when airlines let broke students travel the world?)

Anyway, given that mea culpa, the show's intimate relationship to you over the last few months has allowed me to gain valuable insights into your mental health and states of mind. I'm proud of the open dialogue we've had about tailoring group or individual psychological support at home for the 40 percent of you that remain overly anxious or depressed. Based on your starting weights, a much higher rate of anxiety and depression and medication use was expected; mood problems were maybe somewhat lower in our group as the casting process searched for gregarious, "up" personalities—however, it's interesting to note that even this intense screening process was not able to screen out persons with significant depression.

Are You Running Toward Your Goal or Away from Something Else?

If you're running away from problems, explore every resource to get your mind healthy. Your body will thank you. Don't ever scrimp on health care, either mental or physical—that is priority number one.

If you're running toward your goal, make sure you're properly equipped. Use your exercise, food, and thought journals to continue your exercise and food "education," to hone your coping skills, to identify "bad-habit" triggers, to learn to shake off one-meal setbacks, and reenergize your resolve. When you're screwing up—when eating out or travel or life begins to overwhelm you—go back to the basics; get back on a rigorous exercise, meal, and snack schedule in your controlled home environment.

Set short-term goals: I'm going to work out twice today and plan ahead for two of my snacks to be anabolic shakes; I'm going to eat five different-colored vegetables, three fruits, and no processed carb servings. Set intermediate goals: I'm going to learn to play tennis with my kids; I'm going to run a 10K or marathon. Finally, set long-term goals: I'm going to feel, look, and be like someone 10 years younger than my chronological age and set an example for my kids, then visualize your success!

If you're working out for life, life tends to work out for you. If you're working out solely for looks or to make somebody else happy, it's a much iffier proposition.

Next week, the ultimate motivator—the halftime speech I wrote for Al Pacino, which Oliver Stone rudely edited (imagine the nerve of this guy who only won two Academy Awards), only using a portion in the final cut of his movie, *Any Given Sunday*.

THE WOW! ℞—WEEK TWENTY-ONE

Stay with the Halftime Agenda

Dr. Huizenga Recap—Week Twenty-One

Week Twenty-One Totals for the 36 State Home Contestants:

Average week twenty-one weight loss: women, 2 pounds (0.9%); men, 2 pounds (0.9%)

Average weight loss: women, 52 pounds (21.2%); men, 82 pounds (24.1%)

Last week, out of the blue, an ex-Raider player e-mailed me an intense five-minute workout video—the soundtrack being the halftime football speech of *Any Given Sunday*—part of which, unbeknown to him, I'd written years before. Still more of a coincidence, when I reheard the words, parts of the speech drew parallels to our current 36 home team weight-loss struggles.

Odd as it may sound, there are many similarities between couch-potato participants in fat-loss contests and pro football players. One, of course, is size; but two and three are determination and perseverance. Pro football players, elite male athletes, get and stay in condition by doing up to four all-out hours a day in summer "two-a-days" and keep coming back for more. *Biggest Loser* ranch contestants, both men and women, many who'd never played a high school sport, are getting in condition by doing up to four all-out hours a day in summer "two-a-days" and keep coming back for more. It's said that once the football season begins, to varying degrees, every starter plays hurt. *The Biggest Loser* ranch participants averaged two significant overuse injuries over their first three months of daily exercise and, like oft-injured footballers, had to "play through" injuries and rely on professional athletic trainers and sports doctors for rehab treatments.

Fortunately, in the current 36 home group whom I've instructed to "only" work out 2 to 2.5 hours a day, the initially observed nagging injury rate has been now lowered dramatically (fourfold!). Still, injuries can occur, so it's crucial for everyone to understand that an injury is not a reason to stop exercise. As I've said before, overuse injuries actually heal more quickly if you keep moving; just back off on the sport/activity that caused the injury and cross-train in a sport/activity that places less stress on the injured area of your body. Why do individuals who continue to exercise in the face of overuse injuries tend to heal faster than those who elect complete rest? Injured muscles and tendons still need some stress to optimally heal (just lower levels of the kind of stress that caused the injury). That's part of the reason why, despite frequent injuries in the initial televised seasons of *The Biggest Loser*, all participants continued nonstop cross-training and were injury free at the show finale.

Year after year, most *Biggest Loser* participants thought I was joking when I'd announce after a month of tough workouts, "You're a professional athlete!" But think about it: A pro athlete is someone who gets paid to entertain fans at live venues or on TV while competing in some sort of physical challenge. NFL athletes may be faster, quicker, stronger, and more coordinated, but as far as willpower and desire, they've got nothing over *Biggest Loser* champions. Actually, the mind-boggling part to me is not that lifelong couch potatoes with 100-plus pounds of excess flab can get so physical so quickly when properly instructed, it's that, without exception, every single obese, morbidly obese, and even beyond morbidly obese contestant (all were first properly screened for prohibitive health problems, of course) was able to quickly ramp up to exhaustive, high-intensity exercise!

The last similarity between our 36 home group and pro athletes—we've got superstars too! Eight women are in position to lose more than 27.5 percent of their weight and lose 75 pounds of fat; three or four are currently in position to do what no prior *Biggest Loser* woman and no other outpatient weight-loss female patient has done over eight months: lose more than 100 pounds of fat (Jen Kersy, the current female world fat-loss record holder on *Biggest Loser-2*, lost 99 pounds of fat!). Eleven of the men are in position to lose more than 30 percent of their weight and over 100 pounds of fat. Pete Thomas' 194 pounds, the current male world fat-loss record, also on *Biggest Loser-2*, will be tough to beat, but records are meant to be broken, and several of the men are currently losing fat at this dizzying pace.

"Do you see those extra inches that are all around (and draped all over) us? It's time we heal (pound of fat by pound of fat) as a team. It just might be the difference between living and dying!"

Check out the entire *Any Given Sunday* halftime speech by Al Pacino online at http://www.youtube.com/watch?v=Wo4tIrjBDkk. Every big star gets a "for your consideration," Oscar-worthy soliloquy, and this was it. Let me freely admit, also, that it was a life highlight to see Pacino speak some of the very words that I wrote with Lisa Amsterdam and Oscar winners Oliver Stone and John Logan.

THE WOW! ℞—WEEK TWENTY-TWO

Stay with the Halftime Agenda

Dr. Huizenga Recap—Week Twenty-Two

Questions and Answers

Question: You gave me a WOW! weight of 139 (what you said I'd weigh if I lost only fat and wanted to end up with a body fat of 25 percent). My doctor told me ideally after my weight loss I should have a BMI of 25 or less. I'm hopelessly confused. Are they the same thing?

Answer: No! Body-fat percentage and BMI are worlds apart. But whew, shuffling these cockamamie numbers around is confusing—for doctors and patients alike! Clearly, you can't judge body composition based solely on weight. A muscular 5'10" woman could be very lean at 180 pounds; a 5' woman would have excess fat at 180 pounds. The body mass index (BMI) can be an indication of your body composition because its formula is based on a person's weight and height (weight [lbs] x 703 ÷ height (in)^2). In medicine, we're taught that a BMI less than 25 is normal, a BMI over 25 and under 30 is overweight, a BMI over 30 is obese, and lastly a BMI over 40 is morbidly obese. In the above example, the lean 5'10" woman has a borderline BMI of 25.8, the 5' woman an obese BMI of 35.

Unfortunately, the BMI index is often misleading. Bo Jackson had the most perfect body I ever examined; he was arguably the best physical specimen ever in pro sports, at 6'1", 240 pounds, with not an ounce

---

Week Twenty-Two Totals for the 36 State Home Contestants:

Average Week-Twenty-Two weight loss: women, 1 pound (0.6%); men, 2 pounds (0.9%)

Average weight loss: women, 53 pounds (21.7%); men, 84 pounds (24.8%)

---

of excess fat. But in his prime, his BMI (32) screamed obesity! Conversely, I commonly see patients, especially women, with low weights and low BMIs in the 20 range with abnormal body-fat percentages in the 40 range—"iceberg obesity." Similarly, when losing weight, the BMI can be more confusing than helpful. Although the BMI goes down with weight loss, it never reflects the quality of weight loss. Are the lost pounds all fat, muscle, bone, water? With the availability of Bod Pods and DEXA scanners, anyone on a diet-only or diet-plus modest exercise weight-loss plan would be well served to obtain serial body-fat measurements to gauge healthy versus harmful types of weight loss. (See Table 9.9.)

An example will bring this to life. You started out "obese," both based on your BMI (30) and your body-fat percentage (40). What might happen if you dropped weight by eating very little, exercising very little, avoiding carbs, and dehydrating in the sauna? During a two-month period, this dieting, dehydrating female could lose 30 pounds: 7 of it fat, 6 of it salt water needed to "service" fat, 17 of it muscle tissue and muscle support fluids, and 0.3 pounds of it bone. Everyone would agree that this is a terrible idea, the muscle mass drops, body-fat percent actually increases to 43 percent, the critical lean intracellular water drops, initiating muscle breakdown signals, but notice the BMI is 25—right at "ideal!"

On the other hand, if you followed The WOW! ℞ for two months, you'd lose the 30 pounds: 27 of it fat, 9 of it now unnecessary "support" fluids for fat, with a net gain of 6 pounds of muscle tissue and muscle-support fluids and no change in bone mass.

Table 9.9 Comparison of Sample
Female Weight-Loss Methods

	Obese	Fad Dieting Dehydrating	WOW! ℞	"Normal"	Iceberg Obesity
Height	5′5″	5′5″	5′5″	5′5″	5′5″
Weight (lbs)	180	150	150	137	121
BMI[a]	30	25	25	23	20
Body Fat (%)	40	43	30	25	40
Fat (lbs)	72	65	45	35	48
Protein[b] (lbs)	4	3	2	2	3
Water[b] (lbs)	7	6	4	3	4
Water[c] (lbs)	12	10	8	6	8
Protein[d] (lbs)	24	19	25	25	16
Water[d] (lbs)	21	16	23	23	14
Water[e] (lbs)	34	25	36	36	23
Bone (lbs)	6	5.75	6	6	5

[a] Weight (lbs) $\times$ 703 $\div$ height (inches)^2
[b] In fat cells
[c] Outside fat cells
[d] In organ/muscle cells
[e] Outside of cells

Here's the payoff: Both the fad dieting dehydrating and The WOW! ℞ women lost 30 pounds and they both lowered their BMI from 30 (obese) to 25 ("borderline normal"). However, in the first example, the body fat increased from 40 percent to 43 percent with a clear deterioration in health, and in the second case the body fat deceased from 40 percent to 30 percent with a clear improvement in health. Similarly, in my practice, I've seen individuals who lose 30 pounds of weight: an in-depth breakdown revealed 10 to 15 pounds were water and muscle—only 20 pounds were hydrated fat. Compare them with the

WOW! ℞ long-term winners, whose first 30 pounds of weight loss were 30 to 40 pounds of hydrated fat. Yes, they lost more fat than weight because they gained 5 to 10 pounds of hydrated muscle and physiologic (healthful) fluid.

That's why I gauge a diet's success based on body-fat changes, not weight or BMI changes. That's also why I stated so emphatically that regular scale weights, BMIs, and body-fat assessments are worlds apart!

THE WOW! ℞—WEEK TWENTY-THREE

Week Twenty-Three Agenda with Adjustments

- Daily exercise as scheduled
- Daily healthy eating as scheduled
- Daily entries in your exercise, food, and thought journals
- Same end-of-week routine

However, include the following adjustments:

When you get within 10 pounds of your WOW! weight, add 100 calories (women) and 150 calories (men) to your daily calorie allotment. Lower your exercise to 9 hours a week (1.5 hours, six days a week)—one third endurance (nonstop aerobic exercise), one third interval training (after a proper 15- to 20-minute vigorous warm-up, 6 to 16 sprints (running, swimming, biking, elliptical trainer, rowing) lasting 10 to 60 seconds followed by 20 to 180 seconds of a slow warm-down (i.e., walking) and one third circuit weightlifting (PPT or other forms of circuit training).

When you get within 5 pounds of your WOW! weight: Add 200 calories (women) and 300 calories (men) to your daily calorie allotment. Lower your exercise to 1.5 hours five days a week. Feel free to emphasize your favorite exercise modality, but you must circuit weight lift at least 45 minutes twice a week. A good starting point might be one third endurance, one third interval training, and one third circuit weightlifting. When you reach your desired WOW! weight, begin the MAINTAIN! Plan (see Week Twenty-Seven, page 270).

Dr. Huizenga Recap—Week Twenty-Three

Remember how hopeless and overwhelmed you felt the first week of The WOW! ℞? Whew! Now the tables have turned. After reviewing your recent photographs, I'm overwhelmed by your new "figures." The 36 State Home Team women have lost an average of 22.4 percent, the men 25.7 percent, and you've got a whole new look. Amazingly—without exercising in plastic sweats, participating in wacky "last-chance" workouts, or fluffing "weight" loss numbers by dehydrating or carb depleting— the 36 State Home Team has pulled into a virtual tie with the original *Biggest Loser*-1 contestants. Believe me when I say you've shown the heart of a championship squad!

When we met during my crash fat-loss seminar, I told you, "Stick to the basics. We can do it." Then you went home and did it. . . on your own. Each of us owes a debt to the original *Biggest Loser* participants who blazed this innovative path, but now you've established credibility of your own, showing millions of other Americans and their doubting doctors that there's a practical, economical, safe, sometimes even enjoyable way to reliably drop dramatic amounts of weight. And that way doesn't depend on live-in boot camps, trainers, constant TV cameras, or prize money. You've given millions of unhealthy individuals an

---

Week Twenty-Three Totals for the 36 State Home Contestants:

Average Week-Twenty-Three weight loss: women, 2 pounds (0.9%); men, 3 pounds (1.1%)

Average total weight loss: women, 54 pounds (22.4%); men, 87 pounds (25.7%)

---

alternative to hocus pocus Internet sites, miracle weight-loss pills, fad diets, and even gastric-bypass surgery.

Bottom line, we came together as a team with an initial goal to achieve our WOW! weights and we're poised to achieve that goal! Now, can we peek into the future for a few seconds? Are you ready for your next challenge? Fat maintenance! A lot of doctors call this stage weight maintenance, but my experience shows they've got it wrong. We need to refer to this end game as fat maintenance, because after tapering off of the aggressive fat-loss segment of The WOW! ℞, many former contestants have been able to gain lean tissue (muscle and water). Therefore, your weight—but not your waist—is allowed to increase a bit.

A slow transformation from the aggressive fat-loss phase to the fat-maintenance phase should begin when you approach your desired weight. Ten of our 36 are circling their WOW! weight and have been schooled on the taper-into-fat maintenance plan. The rest of you still have an average of 30 to 40 pounds to go. Stay focused, with your foot to the pedal. Remember: You have committed a huge amount of time and energy to defeat a common foe. To run a personal best time, you need to push a little harder on the initial lap and on the last lap. So, for the next month, I implore you to work out as intensely and as regularly as possible, 2 hours a day, 6 days a week; count calories and stay at your caloric allotments without fail. And last but not least, I demand that you have the time of your lives doing it! Don't waste a second worrying about anyone else or what could have been or what should have been or bad genes or bad luck or bad vibes or blah-blah woof-woof. Go out and run this last lap as if your life depends on it—because it does—with your chest out proudly, grinning ear to ear, and eyes wide open for the new life awaiting you.

Psychological Corner from Dr. Alexa Altman

Congratulations! Over the past five months you have all proven that sedentary obese individuals can be successful at dramatic fat loss. Every day with continued weight loss, you are reinforcing the internal belief that this is possible and that you are going to hit your WOW! weight.

Let's take a step back and examine what has helped you successfully stay on course. These are the top five psychological factors that I have observed to be most critical for your fat-loss success:

1. *Successful fat losers write or look at goals daily.*
   Stay connected to personal goals. We need direction! Have you ever been in a forest without a map? I have, and I will never do it again. If you don't know where you are going, you will most likely move in circles.
2. *Successful fat losers have developed and nurtured their social net-works.*
   Create or expand support. If our social environment resembles a dry, hot, barren desert, we will have a difficult time growing and developing. We need a rich and fertile environment to grow.
3. *Successful fat losers don't interpret a small slip up as a failure; they get back on the horse right away.*
   Embrace gray thinking. Most of us try to divide our world into nice neat categories and think in black and white, subconsciously attempting to distill overwhelming amounts of information into more manageable bits. I am good or I am bad. The diet is working; the diet doesn't work; I can't tolerate the diet. This type of thinking (i.e., one small mistake means your months and months of effort are an utter failure) is a setup for disaster. In truth, the world is different shades of gray. A small dietary indiscretion or a missed exercise session is not good, it's not desirable, but if it's a relatively isolated occurrence, over the long haul it's a barely noticed blip on life's radar.
4. *Successful fat losers appropriately utilize the medical health-care system.*
   Utilize resources. If I told you that you were about to go on the longest journey of a lifetime, six whole months, you would want to pack your bag and make sure you had enough clothes, water, food, etc. This is an arduous journey. There are no extra points awarded for doing it without your bags packed. Find a health-care team you

---

trust, then use them. If you were having a heart attack, you wouldn't think about going it alone. Your centripetal weight may not kill or disable you as quickly as a myocardial infarction, but statistically speaking, it will get you. It is a paramedic-level emergency.

5. *Successful fat losers appropriately utilize the mental health-care system and seek referrals for medication if indicated.*
Identify problems early. What is getting in the way? Is it emotional eating, depression, anxiety, recent losses, work stress? Do you want to address the big roadblock right in the middle of your path, or continue to walk over and around it?

THE WOW! ℞—WEEK TWENTY-FOUR

Follow the Week-Twenty-Three Agenda with adjustments

Dr. Huizenga Recap—Week-Twenty-Four

E-mail Flagged Urgent:
Dear Dr. Huizenga,

I just weighed myself. . . and that scale was undoubtedly at 177!!! I mean, it may be 178 later as it fluctuates throughout the day, but this morning, there was no ambiguity. . . the scale told me plain as day that I'VE LOST 100 POUNDS!!!!!!!!!!!!!!

I absolutely got tears in my eyes. . . I just cannot believe it! When I went to the open *Biggest Loser* audition in Boston, I wrote on the application that I wanted to lose 100 pounds. . . but at the time that seemed impossible, especially for a nonathletic woman!! I just chose an arbitrary number that I thought sounded big enough to get me on the show!! And then of course when I wasn't selected for the show, I figured it was absolutely impossible!!!!!!!!!!!!!

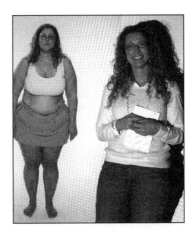

Now two more pounds and I will be at my weight from when I was 15. I have not weighed what I weigh this minute in 12 years! I cannot believe this!!! WHERE DID ALL THE FAT GO??????

VIRGINIA BOURQUE, VERMONT

Congratulations! We're early in the fifth month and already—totally on your own at home—you're a triple-digit loser!!! (P.S. I'm thinking the last pound of fat loss was you hitting that exclamation key!!!!!!!!!!!!!!!!!!!!!) I love your "where-did-all-the-fat-go" question! You probably intended it as a rhetorical figure of speech, but as you can well imagine, I'm all worked up over the scientific and health implications.

When fat "burns up" in the body, it transforms into gas, water, stored energy, and heat. One pound of typical fat combines with 2.75 pounds of oxygen to form 2.66 pounds of carbon dioxide, 1.09 pounds of water, plus lots of energy—about 40 percent stored in our body for future use as ATP (high-energy adenosine triphosphoric acid bonds)—the rest is released into the atmosphere as heat.

You lost 100 pounds of fat, so you sucked down an extra 275 pounds of oxygen (if you extracted every drop of oxygen, you'd have breathed in about an extra 20,000 cubic feet of air), then you breathed out an extra 266 pounds of carbon dioxide (yes, this is air pollution). You also urinated an "extra" 109 pounds of water down the drain. And the

---

Week-Twenty-Four Totals for the 36 State Home Contestants:

Average Week-Twenty-Four weight loss: women, 2 pounds (1.2%); men, 3 pounds (1.1%)
Average total weight loss: women, 57 pounds (23.4%); men, 90 pounds (26.5%)

350,000 "extra" calories you burned? Enough to fuel a run from Los Angeles to New York—except for the fact that some carbs need to be metabolized simultaneously to enable all this fat to burn.

Questions and Answers

Question: I've now got some loose skin on my arms and lower abdomen. Help! Suggestions?

Answer: First off, skin has an amazing ability to stretch and later retract—witness a woman's waist with full-term twins. After the babies are delivered, the abdomen circling the belly button is normally "doughy" for many months, before fully firming up over the ensuing year. That said, there are limits. The abdomen can expand only so much for only so long before permanent damage sets in—visible purplish stretch marks or post- weight-loss/overweight pregnancy floppy, droopy skin. What's the point of no return? It's based on an individual's genetically endowed skin elasticity, which decreases with age, sun damage, cigarette use, length of time stretched, and rapidity of weight gain. No creams have been shown to ameliorate or prevent the aftereffects of skin stretching. As an aside, aging adults shrink inches in height, in part due to bone loss, further contributing to "extra" abdominal skin. Exercise (which prevents bone loss) is an anti-loose-skin, anti-wrinkle potion.

Some recommendations:

- Include calcium and vitamin D in the diet, along with weight-bearing exercise to maintain height, posture, and bone mass.

- Avoid excessive sun (any amount that causes redness and peeling).

- Do not smoke.

- Avoid excessive pregnancy-related weight gain.

- If stretch marks are your only problem, leave them alone. For the most part, these reddish-purple lines, which tend to form around the breasts, shoulders, hips, and, of course, the abdomen, even in normal-weight individuals who have sudden growth spurts, will fade with time to unobjectionable normal skin tones.

For your post-weight-loss drooping skin:

- Wait at least one year to give your skin an opportunity to retract.

- Wait at least one year to assess the physical and psychological impact of the excess skin.

- Do not consider surgical correction if you plan to lose additional weight. Dieting off the last drop of abdominal fat may come with a cost—looking gaunt. Vigorous exercise is the only way to possibly circumvent this phenomenon.

- Wait until your weight is perfectly stable on the fat maintenance plan. Don't proceed surgically until you've stayed at the same weight for at least six months in a row.

- Consider "body contouring"—the last frontier of plastic surgery procedures—with caution: Only consult board-certified plastic surgeons, preferably with extensive experience in post-weight-loss skin-tightening surgery. Ask to see before and after photographs of other people who have had the procedure with this physician and, if possible, call patient references that can be provided. And absolutely get two opinions.

- Abdominal and hip liposuction may be warranted for residual small pockets of fat where further fat loss would excessively lower body fat and make your features gaunt. Remember, however, even aggressive liposuction rarely removes more than 10 pounds of tissue, of which, at most, only two-thirds is fat.

- "Total body contouring" procedures range from standard

outpatient tummy tucks to two-stage lower, then upper-body lifts requiring up to a week in the hospital.

• The real shocker? Fat removed en masse via plastic surgery may make you "thinner" but not necessarily healthier. As compared to an equal amount of fat lost through exercise with caloric restriction, fat physically cut out is not "recognized" by the body. Fat cut out has no discernable ability to lower glucose, blood pressure, or cholesterol!

Question: When I work out especially hard, my shirts are drenching wet. Does this mean I'm burning more calories?

Answer: Sorry, you can't rate the intensity of a workout based on the volume of your sweat. You know that even while sitting perfectly at rest in a hot, humid room, you can perspire through every stitch of clothing. Conversely, you could run a world-class marathon time on a see-your-mouth-breath morning and not visibly sweat a drop (it evaporates before you can see it). Similarly, you could perform an exhausting swim in cool water and never sweat, and, if the water was cool enough, you'd actually be freezing cold during maximal intensity exercise.

True, all things being equal, you'll sweat more during more intense exertion, but you'll also sweat more if you're male, have eaten recently, are in higher ambient temperature and humidity, are more fit, are more hydrated, when there's less of a breeze, the less your exercise involves movement (outdoor biking and running versus stationary biking and treadmilling), the heavier the clothing you're wearing, the more layers of clothing, the tighter the clothing, the more muscular you are, or the fatter you are. And outdoors you'll sweat more in dark-colored clothing. This was a very real problem I faced back in the glory days of the Raiders football team when we wore black jerseys, both home and away during sweltering summer afternoons—and still won week after week. And you'll sweat more in dry clothing than in wet workout gear (heat loss via evaporative cooling is far more efficient with a soaked shirt).

One thing you can estimate from sweating: the relative calorie burns from different parts of your workout. For instance, I did a hard hill run early this morning in the dark for 45 minutes and felt moderately warm and sweaty despite 65°, low-humidity conditions. I then immediately began my circuit weightlifting routine in my outdoor patio gym and noted about 10 minutes later that I was a little chilly. My shirt wasn't dripping wet and a cool breeze had not just begun. I can therefore infer that my circuit-training regime burns fewer calories per unit time than my hill running.

THE WOW! ℞—WEEK TWENTY-FIVE

Follow the Week-Twenty-Three Agenda with adjustments

Dr. Huizenga Recap—Week-Twenty-Five

WOW! You've worked your derriere–and your waist—off. Now, step back, turn slowly, and stare for a minute into a full-length mirror. Unbelievable. . . right? In less than six months, a remarkable metamorphosis! You 36 State Home Team women have, on average, morphed from 243 to 185 pounds, with an average 37 pounds to go until your 148-pound

---

Week-Twenty-Five Totals for the 36 State Home Contestants:

Average Week-Twenty-Five weight loss: women, 1 pound (0.6%); men, 2 pounds (0.7%)

Average total weight loss: women, 58 pounds (23.8%); men, 91 pounds (27.0%)

WOW! weight. So you've shed 61 percent of all your excess fat. You home team men have morphed from 339 to 248 pounds, shedding approximately 71 percent of your excess fat, leaving on average 38 pounds to go until your 210-pound WOW! weight.

It's breathtaking to watch your confidence, control, and enthusiasm grow even more than your waists and hips have shrunk. A physical and emotional transformation of this scope is heretofore unreported in modern medicine. You all qualify for the *Guinness Book of World Records.* You've lost more weight, gained more energy, and extended your lives during this six-month span more than any other recorded outpatient group on a regular food diet!

What I'm especially excited about, based on a sampling of your peers, is that unlike current popular diets, you've lost weight without sacrificing lean tissue. As I'll explain next week, that could pay huge dividends in the future.

For those of you already circling your WOW! weight, you've added 200 calories (women) and 300 calories (men) to your daily allotment and lowered your exercise to nine hours a week—a one-hour, six-days a-week (intense aerobics) in the morning and an hour three afternoons a week (intense circuit training). With this approach, you will gradually taper to a calorie intake that maintains your "body weight" while continuing to lose some excess fat and begin to emphasize body shape (muscle gain) over the next several months. I'll explain these points in detail in an upcoming week. But right now I need to go research an outrageous question just e-mailed to me; the implications of this question are so startling, it has brought my medical office to a grinding halt!

THE WOW! ℞—WEEK TWENTY-SIX

Follow the Week-Twenty-Three Agenda with adjustments

Dr. Huizenga Recap—Week Twenty-Six

Questions and Answers:

Question: Some doctor was on *Oprah* today and he said that for every 35 pounds you lose, your penis grows an extra inch! Any truth to this? I was watching the show with my mom and she kind of looked over at me, 'cause she knows I've dropped just under 100 pounds, as if to say, "You stud! Be careful, you could really hurt someone!"

Answer: There is definitely some truth to this. But to understand, let's go back to sex anatomy 101. Interestingly, the penis is one of the few body parts with no subcutaneous fat—if you gain a ton of weight, none goes to the penis. Similarly, if you lose a ton of weight, the penis doesn't shrink. However, one of the choice spots for fat to accumulate is the suprapubic fat pad that sits smack dab on top of the pubic bone.

When you gain weight, because the base of the penis is firmly attached via a strong ligament to the pubic bone, the thicker the suprapubic fat roll, the smaller the visible flaccid (much more than the erect) penis will be. Ultimately, men may develop a pannus of fat that completely obscures the penis (despite the fact that the absolute—albeit buried—penile size has not changed one iota).

The reverse occurs when men lose weight. If an inch of the suprapubic fat pad is absorbed, the visible portion of the penis may enlarge by as much as an inch. In a brief survey, I determined that approximately half of the male participants and/or their significant others had noted moderate size increases.

Taking a mathematical approach, I looked at the participants' rate of waist shrinkage and calculated that males needed to lose an average of 50 pounds on The WOW! ℞ to drop a one-inch rim of waist fat (in other words, to decrease their abdominal radius by one inch). This translates to needing to drop about 70 pounds in usual fad diets,

---

Week-Twenty–Six Totals for the 36 State Home Contestants:

Average Week-Twenty-Six weight loss: women, 0 pounds (0.2%); men, 1 pound (0.5%)

Average total weight loss: women, 58 pounds (24.0%); men, 93 pounds (27.4%)

---

where only 60 to 70 percent of the total weight lost is fat. On the other hand, midabdominal fat is the first fat to go; suprailiac and suprapubic fat appear to be a bit more resistant. Specifically, male participants had to lose about 140 pounds to lose an inch layer of fat over the front hipbone (anterior iliac crest). It remains uncertain just how much weight needs to be lost to visually elongate the penis an inch (by shrinking the suprapubic fat pad down a full inch), but it appears higher than 35 pounds, probably in the range of 40 to 60 pounds for those on The WOW! ℞, 50 to 100 pounds for those on a regular diet losing relatively more muscle, bone, and water.

Of note: Please be aware that large suprapubic fat deposits may have sexual-satisfaction ramifications in a woman too; suprapubic fat may negatively impact her partner's depth of penetration.

THE WOW! ℞—WEEK TWENTY-SEVEN AND BEYOND

The MAINTAIN! Plan

Establish your MAINTAIN! weight—it can either be your weight at the end of six months on The WOW! ℞ or your original WOW! weight. Ideally, repeat a body composition analysis once you've reached your WOW! weight to see if your muscle mass has increased (hopefully) or decreased (muscle will shrink if it's understimulated and/or underfed) and then recalculate your RDEE and WOW! weight.

- Establish your MAINTAIN! waist—tape-measure parallel to the floor at the belly button, at the end of a breath out.
- Establish your MAINTAIN! rear-end size—purchase the tightest pair of jeans you can squeeze into as your "waist-butt" MAINTAIN! body suit—in indelible ink on inner waistband of pants clearly write "MAINTAIN!" with today's date.

MAINTAIN! Exercise

- One to 1.5 hours of your favorite vigorous exercise five days a week (or 1.5 to 2 hours four days a week). Rotate between intense endurance, interval, and circuit training. (It's okay to emphasize one type, but never totally ignore the other types of conditioning.)
- Individuals with "iceberg" obesity (low BMIs, high body-fat percentage) need to dedicate at least 50 percent of their workouts to weightlifting.
- If possible, tack on one or two additional hours of active family weekend outings such as hiking, tennis, basketball, or skiing.

MAINTAIN! Nutrition

Keep the appetite naturally in check by starting each meal eating the satiating core WOW! ℞ foods:

- Two (women) to three (men) fruit portions—rotate colors compulsively—every day.
- Four (women) to six (men) vegetable portions—rotate colors compulsively—every day.
- Three (women) to four (men) whole-grain/high-fiber servings every day.
- Three (women) to five (men) skinless chicken or turkey every week; four fish portions (low-mercury fish) every week; occasional lean red meat.

- Two (women) to three (men) portions of nonfat milk, yogurt, cottage cheese, or calcium/vitamin D–fortified soy milk every day.
- One portion of healthy fat (in addition to fish): olive oil, nuts, avocado every day; two eggs every other day.
- An anabolic shake or protein-carb facsimile immediately after exercise.
- Wait at least 20 minutes after dinner before considering dessert.

MAINTAIN! Group Support

- Partner with a "sponsor" and send in "payday" weights on the 1st and 15th of every month.
- Help others who are struggling.
- Consult with your medical team if major problems occur.

MAINTAIN! Body Composition

- Weigh yourself weekly on a calibrated scale.
- Put on your baseline "MAINTAIN!" jeans weekly, if you're not already wearing them—and see if they still fit, or if adjustments are needed in your maintenance routine.
- Measure your waist monthly.

MAINTAIN! Self-Monitoring

- **Grand Slam**—You lose weight or stay at your WOW! weight.
- **Home Run**—Your weekly weight is within 5 pounds of baseline.
- **Strike One**—Your weight exceeds baseline by 5 pounds. *Strike One Adjustments:* Weigh yourself each day; journal exercise time and intensity; consume no alcohol or processed carbs. If you've been doing intense weight work and your waist circumference hasn't changed (you can still button up your skintight jeans), readjust your "maintenance weight" up 5 pounds and remove the strike.

You're doing superbly! Your increased weight is muscle!

- **Strike Two**—Your weight exceeds baseline by 7.5 pounds. *Strike Two Adjustments:* Increase exercise to 90 minutes each day; count calories (aim for RDEE × 1.2); journal exercise and diet; if applicable, seek help for depression/alcoholism/ bingeing.
- **Strike Three**—Your weight exceeds baseline by 10 pounds. *Strike Three Adjustments:* Return to the full WOW! ℞ until you again reach baseline weight: calorie count with calorie allotment (RDEE × 0.8); exercise twice a day (10 to 12 hours per week); continue strict exercise and food journaling; repeat front/side photos.

Dr. Huizenga Week Twenty-Seven (Six-Month) End-of-the-Line Recap—Fat Maintenance

Bravo! How good does it feel to finally have this six-month marathon tucked securely under your belt?

You're all fit! You're all eating much healthier (except for a few recent holiday functions, but let's just keep that between us). You're all thinner; many of you are down to your WOW! weights. You've visibly transformed more than could be expected with gastric-bypass surgery—your weight loss is comparable, but your exercise pump, extra muscle, and bone maintenance gives you a distinct cosmetic advantage. And the insides of your brains have changed even more—you're all more energetic, happier, smarter, and self-confident. You're all exercise and diet success stories.

But are you ready for the question? The one you'll hear over and over for the rest of your life?

"How much weight have you regained?"

I'd love nothing more than to heartily congratulate every last one of you and wish you many happy returns. I'd love to be able to tell you to return to your lives invigorated, energized, and refocused, and say that all the tough battles have been waged and won.

Unfortunately, no truly meaningful life transformation is that easy.

THE FINAL STATISTICS!

Six-Month Totals for the 50 Representative Obese and Morbidly Obese Folks from Every State*

Home Contestants (21 women, 15 men)

Average total weight loss: women, 59 pounds (24.2%); men, 95 pounds (27.9%)

Top individual weight loss: woman, 102 pounds (44%); man, 146 pounds (41%)

Lowest individual weight loss: woman, 32 pounds (13%); man, 55 pounds (15%)

Number of participants who lost more than 100 pounds: 11

Number of participants who lost more than 35% of their total weight: 8

Boot-Camp Contestants (7 women, 7 men)**

Average total weight loss: women, 69 pounds (28%); men, 117 pounds (33%)

Top individual weight loss: woman, 103 pounds (39%); man, 173 pounds (43%)

Lowest individual weight loss: woman, 34 pounds (13%); man, 67 pounds (17%)

* The twelve alternates who were sent home with no exercise or diet instruction—but were equally overweight—on average gained a small amount of weight. One of the 62 choose not to participate.

** Approximately each week, one boot-camp contestant was voted off to continue his or her weight loss at home, so that several contestants were at the boot camp for less than a month; four contestants made it all the way until the end of the live-in boot camp, which was four months into the show.

And major weight loss is no exception.

There's a little "fat-maintenance" room tucked deep inside the brain with a roly-poly guard outside holding a rusted key. It turns out that this maintenance man is one vengeful guy. The vast majority of people who lose a large amount of weight regain it all—or, commonly, rebound and become even heavier—within a few years. The details of this backslide are sketchy. There are few, if any, medical studies of people who have lost *Biggest Loser* quantities of weight. The 95 percent rate of weight regain repeatedly quoted in the media was actually the result of a 1959 study of 100 people. More recent analyses, based on random telephone interviews, indicate that the two- to five-year failure rate may be "only" 80 percent—although, because most of us hang up after the first irritating phrase of a telemarketing pitch, this method may not provide the best scientific data.

Bottom line, no other rigorously evaluated home-regular food weight-loss study has ever documented fat loss approaching that of this elite group—hence, there's virtually no precedent to allow us to predict the future. One study compared a rigorous six-month 500-calorie-per-day diet (starting with meal replacement packets and, after four months, switching to regular food plus diet pills) with around three hours of exercise a week to the now popular lap-band weight-loss surgery. At six months both groups had lost around 14 percent of their body weight; at two years (after the surgery and start of the diet), the group on the stringent diet had substantial backsliding and was down to merely 5 percent weight loss, while the surgical group (with additional significant diet and exercise counseling) had actually lost more weight, with a 20 percent loss.

A couple of brief observations: First, the diet tried in this particular study, like so many others with minimal exercise and "artificial food," was, as I've previously explained, destined to fail. Secondly, "weight loss" from a surgical manipulation affecting satiety (compared to weight loss from an exercise-based program) is less beneficial to your overall health on many different levels. The main positive for surgical weight-loss procedures is that they induce 20 percent-plus weight loss, and, long-term, patients keep off over half the weight—far better than any previously studied medical diet. The big negatives are the potentially life-threatening and expensive risks of surgery, a less-healthy type of weight loss (more lean tissue, less fat lost) and lower fitness longevity benefits.

Preliminary information on the 85 *Biggest Loser* participants before this season's 62-person group reveals:

- On average at one year after the finish of their respective seasons, the 64 TV contestants have maintained 78 percent of their end-of-TV-show weight loss (68 percent if you assume the 10 contestants that I couldn't track down regained back all their weight).
- The 21 alternate participants, who were sent home with no instructions, gained 1.3 percent of their weight during this same interval.
- Despite men having a clear advantage over women during the "fat-loss" phase, women appeared to do better at weight maintenance. They maintained 86 percent of their end-of-TV-show weight loss compared to the men's 70 percent (but almost all of the contestants I couldn't track down were women, which could possibly attenuate some of the women's advantage).
- Part of the reason the women appeared to maintain weight loss better is that 30 percent of the females, compared to only 8 percent of the males, actually lost more weight after the TV show finale.
- The first *Biggest Loser* season participants (12), with the longest follow-up so far, are maintaining approximately 90 percent of their end-of-TV-show weight loss at both the one- and two-year marks (no two-year follow-up of two of the participants).

The successful fat-loss maintainers:

- Exercised on average nine hours a week—four hours of vigorous cardio, three hours of vigorous circuit, and two hours of walking level exercise.
- Didn't count calories, but continually mentally monitored what they ate.

The participants who regained 50 percent or more of their weight loss (seven females, four males):

- Exercised on average only about 3 ½ hours a week (1 hour vigorous, 1 hour circuit training and 1 ½ hours moderate).
- Depression, alcohol intake, and increases in TV viewing were risk factors for weight regain.
- The overall *Biggest Loser* participants' weight loss—given dour assumptions about the contestants I couldn't reach one year after the finale—is about 20 percent—comparable to gastric band weight-loss surgery at roughly the same follow-up time; but the *Biggest Losers* had less morbidity and superior cosmetic and disease-prevention results.
- The impressive energy, mood, and relationship benefits noted at the finale continued though the first year of fat maintenance.
- The greater the dehydration that was seen in the end-of-show physical exams, the greater the difficulty in maintaining weight. (Remember, again, that weight and BMI are not good health indexes.) If your final weight reflected 10 pounds of salt and water depletion and then you put on an additional 15 pounds of muscle, your weight could go up 25 pounds, while your waist circumference and total body fat remained unchanged—this is the story I've gotten from several male contestants.

So what's a big loser supposed to do?

Stay Smart

You're an obesity survivor. You'll need to do things differently for the rest of your life!

Remember, anyone can lose weight. All it takes is a short-term commitment requiring short-term behavioral changes. Hundreds of different fad and doctor diets—from liquid protein. . . to low fat. . . to low carb. . . to low calories. . . to eating 800 calories per day of only fast food—result in short-term drops in weight.

Long-term fat maintenance is a totally different animal. Never has diet alone been shown to work. Keeping fat off requires seismic life changes: permanent exercise adaptations, a modest list of dietary concessions, and constant self-monitoring. Fortunately, we now have the benefit of experience to help us through the rough patches.

Understand the Science

As you lose weight, your calorie needs decrease; it takes less energy to walk, run, and stand up. For example, if you drop your weight by a third, from 240 to 160 pounds, the gross caloric expenditure of walking four miles per hour would also decrease by a third, from 554 to 363 calories. Worse, if some of this big weight loss is muscle—you face a double whammy. Then even your resting caloric needs will be decreased (remember weight lost from popular commercial plans is typically two-thirds fat, a third lean tissue). Most people make a fatal mistake when responding to this metabolic downshift: They attempt to eat less instead of exercising more.

But you are in a unique position. For starters, you gained muscle in the face of a big weight loss. This is nothing short of amazing! Secondly, you're in shape! So you can burn more calories at rest and during exercise compared with peers of similar weight.

Stay Aware

Do what the long-time big losers seem to be doing. A voluntary national registry exists for dieters who have maintained a 30-pound voluntary weight loss for at least one year. Because it's not a random sample, it can't be used to predict your odds of keeping weight off, but we can glean real life wisdom from their success stories:

- They eat low-fat diets.
- They rarely skip breakfast.
- They're aware of total calories consumed.
- They are consistent with their diets, even on weekends and holidays.
- They work out at least an hour a day.

What's a Minimum Volume of Exercise for Weight Maintenance?

Five vigorous workouts per week appear to be the basement number for weight maintenance. A 200-pound person should shoot for an extra 600 calories per workout over his or her resting metabolic rate of about 100 calories per hour, or around 700 calories per workout. Sample workouts include:

- 30 minutes of running at 8 miles per hour (mph); jogging at 6 mph up a 10 percent incline; biking at 20 mph; competitive swimming; intense rope jumping; or stair jogging

or

- 60 minutes of jogging at 5 mph; walking at 4 mph up a 6 percent incline; tennis, singles biking at 13 mph; freestyle swimming; vigorous circuit weightlifting; stair walking; or mountain backpacking

or

- 90 minutes of walking at 4 mph; walking at 3 mph up a 5 percent incline; low-impact aerobics; tennis, doubles; pushing a power mower; disco dancing; or jogging on a trampoline

or

- 2 hours of walking at 3 mph; moderate calisthenics; moderate weightlifting; Pilates; or leisurely biking at 10 mph

or

- 4 hours of stretching; yoga; or sex (hey, I swear this stuff has been studied and reported in medical textbooks.)

Feel free to mix and match the above activities. For instance, 30 minutes of vigorous circuit weights, plus a 3-mile brisk walk (45 minutes at 4 mph) also burns the extra 600 calories. If you decide to work out just four days a week, increase the exercise workout times or intensities accordingly (an extra 750 calories per workout). You could do this by adding an extra 15 minutes to a 60-minute "600" workout or an extra 20 to 25 minutes to a 90-minute workout.

- If they maintain their muscle mass, their resting metabolic rates do not go down.
- The longer the weight loss is maintained, the greater the chances of long-term success keeping it off.
- Successful weight maintenance gets easier with time, but these folks still have to work hard with diet and exercise 20 years after losing weight.
- The number of those who have achieved long-term success who originally lost the weight on a low-carb diet is quite low.

Stay Fit

For long-term success, exercise is your best ally. At worst, your body is neutral to regular workouts. At best, you get an addictive endorphin high. On the other hand, low-caloric diets eventually turn on you. The body is hard-wired to combat famine at all costs, so voluntary caloric restriction can rarely, if ever, be maintained for more than a few months to a year. Making matters worse, our brains have not evolved to regulate appetite in sedentary individuals—consequently, most sedentary individuals in a fast-food world are destined to overeat.

Yes, I know what some of you are saying. You already know my philosophy: When it comes to exercise, more is better. So if the spirit moves you to exercise more, please, do it with my blessing. However, overtraining is a consideration when you increase exercise, especially the intensity, and you might notice drops in your performance and mood.

Stay Regular

Continue with your regular exercise, meal and sleep schedule. If you decide to work out four, five, or six days per week, try your best to do it at the same time each day and skip the same days each week (for instance, Wednesday and Sunday), thus staying with your routine. Believe it or not, when you (and everyone at home and at work) know exactly when you'll be working out (this week, this month, or a year from now), it frees up exercise time and reinforces the fact that exercise is as important as other necessary activities in your life. The good news: All of you have prioritized; you've made time in your busy schedules for exercise. Where did you get the time? Ironically, the lifestyle changes you initiated because of a television show have resulted in your watching far fewer hours of TV! The first 85 *Biggest Loser* participants watched TV on average 11.5 hours less per week, almost identical to the increased number of exercise hours. More importantly, these tendencies persisted. Television viewing remained significantly lower than baseline levels even a year after the show finished.

Stay regular with your diet too. Your core nutrition should include lean protein sources (fish, fowl, occasional lean red meat, beans, and low-fat milk products), fresh fruits and vegetables with most, if not all, meals, and beneficial fats (olive oil, avocado, nuts). Do not restrict any fruits or vegetables! Whole-grain products in moderation are okay. The emphasis will still be on the good you should eat rather than the junk you shouldn't.

Stay Vigilant

As I've said before, I don't give a damn what you weigh! I do care deeply about your body fat, especially the excess amount residing in your abdomen. Therefore, you need to monitor your waist size and rear-end size. Weight, though clearly not a reliable health index in athletes (yes, that's you now!) is still a simple parameter to follow, so we'll check a weekly calibrated scale weight. If your weight increases due to water or muscle, your maintenance jeans should still fit and that's good! If your waist size expands, that's always bad (except temporarily for a day or two, in the face of female hormonal cycles, a whopper of a meal, or really bad gas).

Stay Suspicious

It was distressing that only a handful of the many young participants I diagnosed with diabetes, prediabetes, or hypertension were aware of their medical conditions. Worse yet, many had the "metabolic syndrome," a grouping of blood pressure, lipid, and centripetal fat excesses that together predict a much, much higher risk of medical disasters than just blood-sugar problems alone. If your stomach bulges out, don't stick your head in the sand. The odds you have a disease affecting your longevity is markedly elevated.

Troubleshoot

Problems will inevitably arise. Your success depends in large part on your ability to adjust to personal crisis, injuries, and plain old down days.

You can follow the currently popular maxim, "Don't sweat the small stuff." But if you start veering off track, you must possess a contingency plan—like the MAINTAIN! plan—to self-correct and get moving again in a positive direction. Never underestimate your appetite. Food gives you life, but today's packaged products and fast food, especially those with refined (processed) carbohydrates and added sugar, put you at special risk. Continue to avoid them! Overeating and drug addiction have many similarities: cravings, triggers, binges, intense pleasurable highs— and relapses, guilt, remorse, and withdrawal. You are a food addict who managed to kick the habit for the last few months, but must still battle junk-food urges—one day at a time.

"Infecting" Others Can Save Lives!

You've all done something quite incredible. But it's just the beginning. Obesity is a contagious disease! If you're way overweight, it appears to shift the perception of "social norms regarding the acceptability of obesity" amongst your friends! We've got to turn this iceberg-bound Titanic around to prevent ever-escalating numbers of needless years of life lost. You've all remarked on the profound influence your incredible weight loss and consistent exercise and nutrition habits have had on your family, friends, and work acquaintances—many of whom had waist overhangs rendered invisible by deep denial. Continue to use your positive spirit, healthful habits, and new bodies to connect with people—and

Table 9.10 Health Assessment for Home State Men (at Six Months)

	Pre	Post	Change	% Improvement
Weight (pounds)	336	243	93	28%
BMI	46	33	13	28%
% Body Fat	45	27	18	40%
Fat (pounds)	149	70	80	54%
Waist (inches)	56	44	12	21%
Hip (inches)	53	44	9	16%
Systolic Blood Pressure (mm of mercury)	148	121	27	18%
Diastolic Blood Pressure (mm of mercury)	94	78	16	17%
Metabolic Syndrome (% participants)	93%	20%	73%	71%
Hypertension (% participants)	93%	27%	66%	71%
Diabetes or Pre-diabetes (% participants)	60%	7%	53%	88%
Snoring Complains (% participants)	73%	13%	60%	82%
Heartburn Complaints (% participants)	27%	0%	27%	100%
Asthma Complaints (% participants)	13%	7%	6%	46%
Cholesterol	166	139	27	16%
Triglycerides (≤ 15)	128	40	88	69%
HDL (good-guy cholesterol) (≥40 desirable)	35	45	-10	28%
LDL (bad-guy cholesterol) (≤100 desirable)	94	80	14	15%
Fasting Glucose (≤100 normal)	113	81	32	28%
Fasting Insulin (≤12 normal)	14	4	10	73%
C Reactive Protein (≤0.3 normal)	0.7	0.3	0.4	54%

Average Years of Life Added   9
(if fitness and weight loss maintained)

Table 9.11 Health Assessment for Home State Women (at Six Months)

	Pre	Post	Change	% Improvement
Weight (pounds)	240	185	55	23%
BMI	40	31	9	23%
% Body Fat	50	37	13	26%
Fat (pounds)	120	70	50	42%
Waist (inches)	51	41	10	19%
Hip (inches)	52	45	7	14%
Systolic Blood Pressure (mm of mercury)	132	117	15	11%
Diastolic Blood Pressure (mm of mercury)	85	77	8	9%
Metabolic Syndrome (% particiants)	38%	5%	33%	87%
Hypertension (% particiants)	62%	20%	42%	68%
Diabetes or Pre-diabetes (% participants)	24%	0%	24%	100%
Snoring Complaints (% particiants)	57%	15%	42%	74%
Heartburn Complaints (% particiants)	43%	0%	43%	100%
Asthma Complaints (% particiants)	19%	12%	7%	37%
Cholesterol	186	162	24	13%
Triglycerides (≤ 15)	83	48	35	42%
HDL (good-guy cholesterol) (≥40 desirable)	55	52	3	-5%
LDL (bad-guy cholesterol) (≤100 desirable)	114	100	14	12%
Fasting Glucose (≤100 normal)	86	77	9	10%
Fasting Insulin (≤12 normal)	8	4	4	55%
C Reactive Protein (≤0.3 normal)	0.9	0.5	0.3	38%

Average Years of Life Added 5
(if fitness and weight loss maintained)

thereby their health. Go out and infect all of America!

Your phenomenal numbers in Tables 9.10 and 9.11 illustrate that The WOW! ℞ is an effective at-home, medication-free way to lower blood pressure and abnormal lipids, reduce asthma, treat depression, essentially eliminate type 2 diabetes, heartburn, snoring, and suppress disease-provoking C-reactive protein. But the best news is on the tables' bottom rows. Amazingly, conservative estimates predict if the Home State participants maintain their fitness and current fat loss, on a statistical basis, they'll live five to nine years longer!

Can you even remotely imagine, if someone came to you and guaranteed adding five to nine quality years to your life, what you would be willing to pay?

Note: Men benefit more than women because they, on a percentage basis, lost more overall fat and more abdominal fat.

Table 9.12 Daily Activity Changes for Home State Men

	Pre	Post	Change
Energy[a]	4	8	4
Depression[b]	4	3	−1
Relationships[a]	6	8	2
Overall life[a]	5	8	3
Exercise (minutes)			
Vigorous[c]	2	63	61
Circuit training[c]	2	22	20
Moderate[c]	3	20	17
Walking[c]	3	18	15
Total exercise (minutes)	**10**	**123**	**113**
TV viewing (minutes)	222	84	−138
Leisure computer (minutes)	79	71	−8

[a]Self-described feelings; 1 to 10 scoring scale
[b]Higher number means greater depression
[c]Minutes a day, 6 days a week

Table 9.13 Daily Activity Changes for Home State Women

	Pre	Post	Change
Energy[a]	4	8	4
Depression[b]	7	2	−5
Relationships[a]	5	8	3
Overall life[a]	5	8	3
Exercise (minutes)			
Vigorous[c]	2	59	57
Circuit training[c]	1	18	17
Moderate[c]	2	9	7
Walking[c]	5	18	13
Total exercise	**10**	**105**	**95**
TV viewing (minutes)	186	54	−132
Leisure computer (minutes)	60	50	−10

[a]Self-described feelings; 1 to 10 scoring scale
[b]Higher number means greater depression
[c]Minutes a day, 6 days a week

Besides the health benefits of exercise, it is an unbelievable brain potion. Male participants (Table 9.12) noted a major boost in energy in the initial months of the program, seemingly more closely tied to fitness than weight loss or changes in sleep. The men found time for 2 hours of exercise a day and an additional 30 minutes of vigorous labor at work or home (yard work) by watching 138 minutes less TV per day, spending 8 minutes less leisure time on the computer, and driving in their motor vehicles 30 minutes less each day.

Female participants (Table 9.13) noted not only the upfront energy enhancement, but also significant mood improvements, again initially seemingly more closely tied to cardiovascular fitness than weight loss or sleep improvements. The women found time for almost 2 hours of exercise a day and an additional 30 minutes of moderate yard or house work—despite all of them being full-time moms and or having full-time jobs by watching 132 minutes less TV and spending 11 minutes less leisure time on the computer each day.

Postscripts

Thirty-five of the original 36 Home State participants gathered in L.A. at the eight-month mark for an emotional graduation ceremony. Here are a few of their poignant graduation essays:

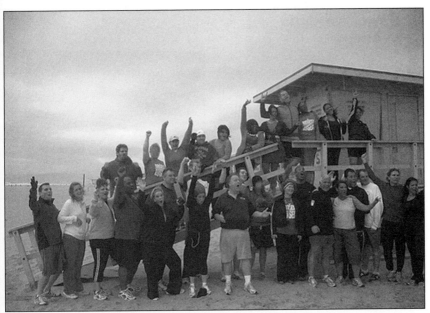

Before graduation, we retraced our first workout route... this time without the medical van following to pickup stragglers... now everyone could run!

— —

After years of promising my family and myself that I was going to lose weight, take care of myself, not die young like my father did, etc., and not following through, I finally made the commitment to keep my word. I told myself I would do everything Dr. H. asked me to do.

It worked. The weight melted off. I averaged about 7 or 8 pounds a week for the first month alone. Very cool! I felt unstoppable. And for the first time in decades, eating well and exercising excited me. About halfway through the weight-loss plan, however, there was a confluence of very negative things that happened in my life. I was experiencing significant marital, financial, and personal problems. It's tough enough to deal with this when you have all of your coping mechanisms at your disposal, but when my biggest one—binge eating—was no longer available, I felt like a boxer punched by Mike Tyson in his prime! I languished for about a month and lost little or no weight for about four to five weeks. After feeling sorry for myself and starting to make sense of what I was faced with at the time, the switch flicked again and I was off and running (no pun intended) again, immediately achieving my highest weekly loss. . . 15 pounds! Very cool!

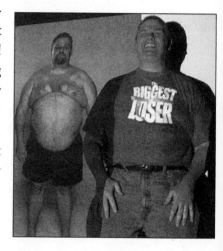

Losing 100 pounds and getting healthy in the face of adversity taught me incredible lessons. I now know what I want out of life. And I now know whom I want around me for the rest of my (now prolonged) life.

WALLY BRESSLER, NEW HAMPSHIRE

Everyone has their own struggles, their own motivations for wanting to lose weight. For me, it was seeing the devastating effects of diabetes. My brother developed adult-onset diabetes. I watched him in intensive care in a diabetic coma. You can't imagine how scary it was when Dr. Huizenga informed me I was pre-diabetic!

That was it. . . I had no choice. But even with this amazing source of motivation, it was still very challenging to lose weight by going from being completely sedentary to exercising twice a day, six days a week. I'm not going to lie, I struggled! I worked a full-time job, had the anguish of dealing with two of my immediate family members being homeless, injured both of my knees, and had a limited budget with which to eat healthy. . . it was overwhelming at times. But keeping small weekly goals and making my exercise my therapy and own personal time to work things

out (both emotionally and physically) kept me going. And when I struggled, I didn't give up. I just kept on doing my best, even if my best wasn't always perfect. I am by no means at my WOW! weight, but I've lost 73 pounds of pure fat and am now confident in my abilities. I have the power to prevent diabetes. My glucose and insulin are now perfectly normal!

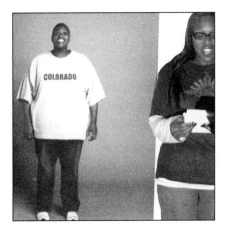

STACIE FARR, COLORADO

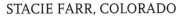

I was always overweight as a child and teenager, but I dreamt of being a professional athlete. The only thing holding me back was my weight. I actually worked my butt off for the opportunity to play baseball and all of my hard work paid off when I played in the Junior College World Series as a walk-on—so much so that my teammates nicknamed me "Rudy" after the inspirational University of Notre Dame football player. My moment of glory: Stealing a base as a pinch runner in the bottom of the 8th inning.

Soon after college, I allowed my health to spiral downward. Not only had I returned to very poor eating habits, but instead of actively playing sports, I had now made it my career to stand on the sidelines coaching sports. There were many nights when I only had time to grab a burger (or three) at the drive-through, and many days when I had the perfect excuse to make a pre-game stop at Dairy Queen for a good-luck milkshake! Nine years of teaching and coaching (and burgers and milkshakes) finally took its toll; my weight ballooned. Unbelievably, I was now morbidly obese.

I tried countless diets; all failed miserably, leaving me even more overweight. Worse yet, failure left me extremely depressed and empty on the inside. Finally, one day, my students challenged me to make a life change. They challenged me to try out for *The Biggest Loser.* I had always challenged my students, so when they threw it back in my face, I knew that I had to try my best.

As a teacher and coach, I know the value of a good education. All of my life, even during my almost-professional athlete days, I never received one iota of input on healthy eating! When I listened to Dr. H. and the other experts talk, I decided not to challenge anything I was taught.

I just followed the program and trusted. When others were saying, "I can't work out two hours a day!," I would say, "I will work out two hours a day!" End result, I successfully dropped 114 pounds of fat. I now run a sub-6-minute mile and recently captured a state and a national racquetball championship. I'm thin on the outside and full of life on the inside. But best of all, I'm able to inspire others again. You know what? The other day, an old college buddy called me *Rudy*!

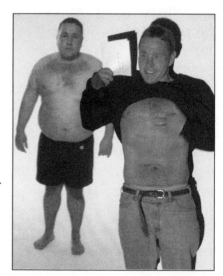

TIM CLAUSEN, DELAWARE

"How on *Earth* did you go from a size 22 to a size 2 in under 8 months?!" That's the question everybody asks.

I know it sounds like magic, but really, the magic is in your commitment to the program. This was the first time in my life I just put my head down and ran. Consistently. Every day. Literally and figuratively. I promised myself I'd finish what I started, and for the first time in my life, I did.

I never called the healthy eating plan a "diet" because I was *never* hungry, loved what I ate, and continue to do so! I never called the workouts *work* because after the first month or so, when the aching finally subsided, exercise actually became fun (when it was over).

Things from Dr. H.'s program that really resonated with me:
1. I needed carbs to work out effectively!
2. I measured everything I ate on a food scale.
3. I wrote down everything I ate. *Everything.*
4. I had Dr. Huizenga's anabolic shakes after working out every day—it helped me retain muscle mass while burning fat.
5. I was creative. I figured out how to replace my old fat-laced enemies with new fresh friends! (Ew! Did I actually just *say* that?)
6. When my workout became comfortable, I changed it up! I always pushed myself. I started out unable to do much, but day after day I showed up at the gym. I did 2.5 hours a day, more than I needed to according to

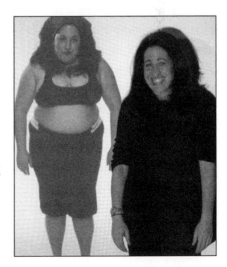

Dr. H., but I was completely horrified by my size!
7. I was consistent.
8. When I fell off the wagon, I didn't kill myself. I just got back to the gym.

Things that really amaze me:
1. I still work out seven to nine hours a week—and actually like it (most of the time)!
2. I've kept all the fat off.

I know it sounds like magic, but really the magic is your mind.
POPPI KRAMER, NEW JERSEY

I am a 15-year veteran police officer. While on routine patrol, August 2005, a car veered into me. I was almost killed. Barely able to move a finger for four months, I watched TV, ate junk food, and gained even more fat—65 pounds, to be exact. One day, flipping channels, a reality TV show caught my attention; it seemed to be talking to me about my weight problems. Miraculously, I was accepted as an at-home contestant!

Dr. Huizenga (better known to many of us as Dr. H.) grabbed my attention and changed my life from the first moment of our weight-loss seminar when he stressed the critical role of exercise. He truly made me realize I needed to lose fat (not muscle or bone or water) and that fat maintenance will be something that I have to pay attention to forever. There is no such thing as a quick fix.

Dr. H.'s WOW! ℞ definitely had its challenges—but no one ever said it would be easy. I had to completely change my lifestyle to make it work. And I had to believe in myself and in Dr. H.'s plan for lifestyle change (rather than a temporary diet like all of the other weight-loss plans out there) and lifelong success. I had to find a way to fit in working out two times a day with my hectic schedule, and the word "vigorous" will always be ingrained into my thought process. I had to work just as hard mentally as physically, and I always tried to remind myself to take it "one day at a time for life's success."

The thanks and admiration I have for Dr. Huizenga will truly be unmeasured. Your program is what I have always searched for (but didn't realize it): A complete lifestyle change. I lost 95 pounds, am a happily married newlywed, am back at work on the force full time, and am maintaining my new lifestyle. Dr. H., your program is what people around the world like me have been waiting for. I can never thank you enough, my friend!

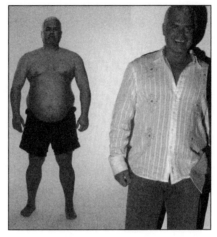

Who would've thought it'd take a devastating accident to turn my life around?

MARK MONACO, MONTANA

Growing up in a rural community in America's heartland, food was a time for celebration! Birthdays, get-togethers, reunions. . . any excuse for eating. . . including "there are children starving in China". . . was good.

I was always the short, fat kid who never got picked for basketball or baseball. I became the life of the party to cover up for my fatness and make people like me—but deep inside I was hurting. After I graduated I opened my own business, got married, had kids, and hurt my ankle (three times). I stopped all physical activities, instead focusing on everyone else but me. I started gaining. . . 200. . . 225. . . 250. . . 275. . . and gaining more. . . 345. . . 375. . . 395. . . 400. . . 'til I hit 410, my all-time high. Miraculously, like a dream come true, I got chosen to compete on *The Biggest Loser*—36 State Home Team.

Now, a year after I started following Dr. H.'s program, I've lost 175 pounds of fat and I feel awesome! I know when I can get outdoors and

be even more active, my last few pounds will melt away and I will offi-
cially hit my WOW! weight. This experience has brought me closer to
my family, friends, and most of all, *me*! I'm a new person. The outside
me finally matches the inside me!

I feel so lucky to be able to make a difference in other people's lives
now. I travel around speaking to anyone willing to listen about the epidemic of obesity. I tell them how
my life was slipping through my
fingers, one French fry at a time. I
tell them that my fat was literally
weighing me down, that I wasn't
able to love, to laugh, and even
truly enjoy food for a *long time*! And
I tell them that thanks to this program, my life is back; my dreams
are now a reality.

JAMIE DEAN LUCAS,
KENTUCKY

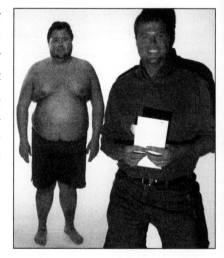

Shhh!. . . don't tell Dr. Huizenga, but I was a "bad" at-home contestant. I was completely motivated, armed with the same powerful
information that you now hold in your own hands—The WOW! ℞
healthy eating and exercise plan. But as a busy professional who frequently worked 12 hours a day, I knew I would have a lot of trouble getting in all of the workouts.

I did my best! I worked out every morning, religiously—waking up
at 5 A.M. every day in order to get a full hard-core 60 minutes of aerobic exercise in (alternate days adding an additional 30 minutes of
strength training if I knew I would miss my evening workout). I managed to do an additional hour of exercise on some days here and there,
but more often than not I would work late and come slumping in my
front door with just enough motivation to fix a healthy dinner before

going straight to bed.

I was afraid that my weight loss wouldn't measure up to the rest of *The Biggest Loser* at-home contestants because I knew that I wasn't doing all of the exercise that I had been prescribed. But you know what? I managed to be one of the top three female fat losers, both mid-season and at the show's finale. I went from a weight of 270 pounds to 162 pounds (a fat loss of 108 pounds!). Perhaps more importantly, I have continued to exercise an hour to an hour and a half six days a week, and have maintained all of my fat loss (actually losing an additional 10 pounds since the show ended!).

Can you *really* manage to work out twice a day, count calories, plan meals and snacks, do extra grocery shopping, and continue to meet family and work expectations? If getting healthy is truly a priority for you, absolutely. But you know what? Even if you cheat a little and only work out vigorously for one hour a day, you can still successfully drop the fat—it just might not be as dramatically quick as the folks on the TV show. Either way, this I promise you: You will get out of this program exactly what you put into it. If you truly stick to The WOW! ℞ and keep your calorie counts where they should be, and truly push yourself to do all of the exercise (and do it at maximum effort rather than lolly-gagging), *you will drop the fat.* I'm living proof.

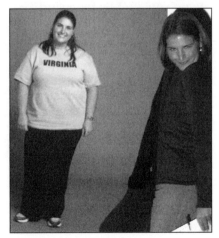

JENNIFER KERNS, VIRGINIA

I've been overweight and underconfident my entire life. I was the cute pudgy/chubby redhead with lots of curls sitting in the back of the class as a little girl, and a fat teen during the 1960s—remember, this was the era of Twiggy! I didn't have boyfriends to take me to dances, or even a date to the prom.

My mother helped me through the hard times, but she taught me two things that backfired. One, eat everything on your plate (of course it was good old-fashioned meat and potatoes with real butter, cream sauces, etc.) and two, be strong and independent because asking for help is a sign of weakness. I was married in my 20s and put on huge amounts of weight with both my pregnancies and then came my emotional eating with my divorce—I never took the weight off. Until *The Biggest Loser* and Dr. Huizenga came along, I never asked for help. I tried many different diets on my own over my 55 years, always losing a little and then gaining it all back plus more.

Finally I had enough! I made the decision to lose weight, meet a good man, play with my grandkids, and show myself I wasn't too old to change my life! By following The WOW! ℞ plan as best I could, I succeeded in dropping 55 pounds. I finally have the freedom—I can walk into any store I want (not just the Big Women's World). I can finally breathe—I jog without my asthma inhaler. I finally stopped all excuses—I fit exercise into my daily life regardless. I finally found love—first I learned to love myself again, then a great guy came into my life and we got married! My last remaining goal is to reach my "WOW!" weight. . . 32 pounds to go. I now know I can get there.

LINDA HOUSEMAN, IDAHO

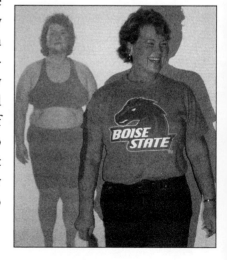

Dr. H. adds: It's amazing what getting fit can do for your love life! In eight months, two women found boyfriends, one woman found a fiancé, one woman found and married her husband, and one man found a fiancée!

I began gaining weight in elementary school. Everyone said not to worry; it was just baby fat; I would outgrow it once I hit puberty. But puberty hit, and I was more overweight! At 14, my parents divorced. Then my fast food/microwave lifestyle really kicked into high gear. After college, I began trying a different diet practically every month: Atkins, South Beach, Weight Watchers, low fat, low carb, Internet diets, book diets, even starvation. Nothing ever seemed to work long term.

Then, one day I weighed myself. The scale couldn't be right?! It showed me at an all-time high of 298 pounds, and I realized that I was about to cross the 300-pound threshold. I made the decision to try out for *The Biggest Loser*. Dr. H.'s WOW! ℞ nutrition and two-a-day workouts really made sense. Everything was simplified: Burn more calories than you take in! I didn't have to count carbs or fat grams, use a heart rate monitor, or any of that other stuff that can muck up the waters. The three big things I concern myself with are: one, calories in; two, vigorous workouts; and three, Dr. Huizenga's anabolic recovery shakes. In the past, I have always been skeptical for one reason or another and therefore not entirely committed. Because of the simplicity of this program, I have finally been able to commit myself 100 percent to something. And I'm seeing 100 percent changes. . . in my body as well as in my mind.

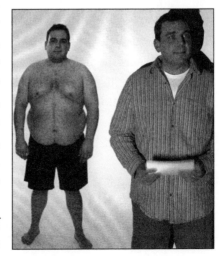

For me, the long-term goal of losing over 100 pounds was too daunting, so I set smaller goals of running races. When I began, I couldn't slowly jog longer than 2 minutes. But within a month, I completed my first 5K. After five months, I had completed five running races and three sprint triathlons. Now, 78 pounds lighter than I was when I started the program, I've never felt more confident that my lifelong bad habits are behind me. And I just completed my first marathon!

Dr. H., you were so right when you said that first day, "You don't have to be thin to be an athlete!"

KEVIN THEIS, WISCONSIN

I was the frustrated "Stuck on Flat Terrain" e-mailer. Let me tell you. . . those 3 weeks—working out and dieting harder than ever and not losing a single pound—almost did me in. Dr. H., you told me losing weight (as compared to fat!) is so much more than calories in and out. . . thankfully, somehow I was convinced to stay the course. Lo and behold, the program worked! I went on to lose 3 pounds a week faithfully for the next three months!!!! And in the process I gained a new love—running! I can't live without it—it's my new happy hour!

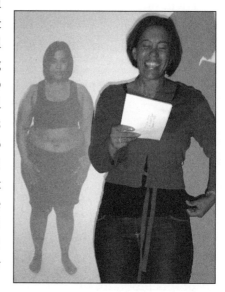

NIKKI MEYERS, OHIO

Dr. H. adds: During this WOW! !weight-loss process, couch-potato, morbidly obese 36 State Home contestants completed three marathons, two half marathons, four triathlons, and participated in over 24 other organized races.

I think my self-perception is still catching up to me. I don't picture myself like I used to be—but apparently I still think of myself as being fatter than anyone around me thinks I am. It's all been so fast, you know? We did a big tournament this last weekend and I was watching the video footage last night. I had done 95 percent of the filming, but we were watching this one part and I didn't recognize one of the players, which was weird, because in spite of there being 70+ players, I thought I knew them all, y'know? But I'm watching it with my wife, and I'm like, who is that guy? It was me!

Seriously. I didn't even recognize myself with the mask and paintball clothes on (I never fit in them before so this was my first time playing in actual paintball jersey and pants. . . *very* cool). Crazy. I ended up watching that clip over and over—just being kind of shocked over it all. Maybe an overreaction? But hasn't it all been so sudden? Do others find looking in the mirror surreal?

MATT MᶜNUTT, MAINE

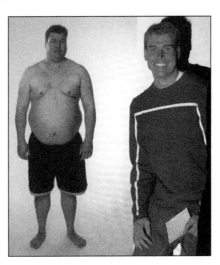

SECTION THREE

HELP IS ON THE WAY

Supplemental material
to facilitate your journey

Chapter Ten

The WOW! ℞ Nutrition Plan

Clean out your refrigerator! Empty your pantry! We're stocking up on your WOW! ℞ "core foods." Start—and maintain—your fat loss by having on hand only the foods you need to eat for success. Of course, I could wag a finger and list the obvious foods you need to detox from—sugary, refined, and saturated fatty foods, and their innocent-appearing kin, artificial sugar and fat—but it's far more productive to focus on the satiating foods that you must eat. In my experience, although temptation in the form of junk food is around every corner, a full stomach considerably reduces its lure.

So resist temptation with preparation: stock your pantry, refrigerator, and freezer with wholesome WOW! ℞ foods, then plan a week's worth of meals in advance. Some of the items that you should have on hand at all times follow.

CORE FOODS PURCHASE LIST

Carbohydrates

Fruit: Stock up on a rotating assortment of colorful (red, yellow, orange, dark green, pale green, violet) fresh and flash-frozen varieties. One serving should be approximately 80 calories, for example: a medium-sized apple or orange, a small (6-inch) banana, 1 cup of diced tropical fruit, or 1 ½ cups diced melon or berries (avoid canned fruit packed in sugary syrups).

Don't be fooled by diet gurus who ban fruits claiming their carbohydrates (fructose) are "obesity-causing sugars." In fact, whole fruit is a dieter's ally—it contains fiber, minerals, vitamins, and antioxidants; sweetness is the bonus! And the sweet fructose actually has a low glycemic index; its absorption and conversion to blood sugar is relatively slow! (The increasing quantity of artificial fructose sweeteners America consumes in drinks and foods is another matter—it raises dire health concerns!)

Avoid dried fruits (not as satiating per calorie as fresh fruit).

No juices (evolution didn't prepare us for liquid food; calorie for calorie they're not as satiating as solid food).

Vegetables: Stock up on a rotating assortment of colorful (red, yellow, orange, dark green, pale green, violet) fresh and flash-frozen varieties; one serving is about ½ cup, or about 15 to 30 calories for most cooked vegetables; winter squash is slightly higher at 40 calories per ½ cup and starchy vegetables (such as peas, corn, beans, and potatoes) are higher still—½ cup will be about 60 to 110 calories—and might be better counted toward the "whole grains" category. Be aware: eating seven servings of beans or potatoes could add up to 600 calories (versus 150 calories in seven usual vegetable servings) and might put you over your calorie limit!

Whole Grains: One serving should be about 80 to 100 calories—for example, ½ cup of cereal (such as Kashi GoLEAN, All Bran, oatmeal), ½ cup of beans, one slice whole-grain bread (or two slices of "light" bread), ½ of a large whole-wheat pita, 2 Wasa Crispbread crackers, or one 6-inch whole-wheat or corn tortilla.

Lean Protein

One serving of lean protein is about 4 ounces raw or 3 ounces cooked; if no scale is available, a cooked piece is approximately the size of a deck of cards. One portion size is 120 to 160 calories, with leaner varieties being lower in calories.

Lean Poultry: Choose chicken and turkey (white meat only, remove skin and other fat).

Fish: Choose from very-low-mercury fish (that children and pregnant women can safely eat three portions of per week), namely, anchovies, catfish, clams, crawfish, herring, mackerel (North Atlantic Chub), Pacific flounder (sanddab), perch (ocean), sardine, scallop, shad, shrimp, sole (Pacific), squid, tilapia, trout (freshwater), whitefish, whiting, and wild salmon (farmed species may contain PCBs—chemicals with negative long-term health effects; when in doubt, don't eat the skin and fatty parts of fish where these chemicals collect). Limit higher-mercury species, like tuna, to once-a-week.

Low-Fat "Red Meat" (in moderation): Choose pork tenderloin, lean red meat "loin" cuts (such as sirloin or tri-tip), or extra lean ground beef (at most two to three portions per week).

Nonfat Dairy Sources: One serving is 1 cup of fat-free milk, yogurt, or soymilk; ½ cup of fat-free ricotta or fat-free cottage cheese; or 1 ounce of hard cheese (light string or cheddar), and is about 80 to 110 calories. Remember, nonfat milk and milk products have healthy carbohydrates, too! Fruit yogurts have added sugar, so make your own fruit yogurt by adding fresh fruit to plain fat-free yogurt.

Vegetarian Protein Sources (in addition to dairy): The following sources are all good vegetarian choices:

- Egg whites or liquid egg substitute (one "lean protein serving" is one cup, 120 calories).
- Whole eggs (up to seven a week are okay, one "lean protein serving" is two large eggs, 140 calories).
- Soy: Edamame (soybeans, when measured with pods, one "lean protein serving" is 1 cup, 150 calories), soy-based veggie burgers (brands differ, but one patty is one "lean protein serving," 130 calories), tofu (3 ounces of firm tofu is one "lean protein serving," 123 calories), plain soymilk (1 cup has 100 calories).

• Beans and legumes: Black beans, garbanzos (chickpeas), kidney beans, lentils, navy beans, pinto beans, split peas ("lean protein serving" is 3/4 cup, 165 calories).

Note: Despite the common misconception that a spoonful of peanut butter is a good source of protein, nuts and nut butters are not high enough in protein to count toward this category—their calories come mostly from fat!

Fat

You will get enough fat in your diet from the other foods you eat (there is fat in most protein and dairy sources), but if you have calories left over, you might choose to add from the unsaturated fats in the following foods:

• Olive oil (extra virgin)—1 teaspoon has 40 calories.
• Canola oil—1 teaspoon has 40 calories.
• Tree nuts such as almonds, walnuts, pecans—watch portion sizes because 1 ounce of nuts has between 160 and 200 calories!
• Avocado—1 ounce has about 45 calories; a whole avocado will often have 300 or more calories, so again, watch portion sizes!
• Extras: Salsa, mustard, spices, nonfat/low-fat salad dressing (choose salad dressings with less than 50 calories per 2 tablespoons).

COUNTING CALORIES

Do you have to write down everything you eat and drink? Preferably within 15 minutes? Yes. Frankly, there's no better way to keep track of your intake and learn the basics of portion size, calories, and nutrition. Sure, it's tedious, time consuming, and sometimes confusing, but seeing every food choice printed out in black and white right in front of your nose is a real eye-opener. Be as accurate as possible with your calorie counts; weigh or measure everything and look up the caloric value of each individual food. Once you get the hang of estimating portion sizes and you begin to lose fat according to schedule, it's reasonable to take shortcuts; read on—page 310 summarizes tricks to save you time.

When you have a concrete calorie count, you're finally in position to take control of your eating. It enables you to differentiate healthy from less-optimal ingredients, to properly balance your nutrition without supplements, and to master portion sizes. Isn't it empowering—after years of relying on food and vitamin manufacturers for information—to finally understand exactly what you're putting into your body? To recognize what foods give you energy, which ones make you feel lousy or push you further up the line toward obesity, cancer, diabetes, and heart disease?

The skinny on why you should keep a food journal:
- Keeping records gives you concrete information.
- It increases awareness of physical versus emotional hunger.
- It alerts you to energizing or fatiguing effects of food.
- It helps problem solve.
- It balances calories.
- It changes self-sabotaging behaviors.

Calorie-Counting Equipment Needed:

- Kitchen scale (accuracy to 0.1 ounce).
- Measuring cups and spoons.
- Food journal (sample in Appendix).
- Calculator. The math can be a bit challenging at first; for instance, how many calories are in a $3/4$ cup portion of cereal if the label lists a 1 $1/4$-cup serving as containing 170 calories? (Or set up your journal on a spreadsheet, where the computer will do some of the arithmetic for you.)

In addition, purchase a pocket-sized calorie-counting book, which includes an index to make finding your food(s) quick and easy; each food's calorie and nutrition facts listed by weight (ounces or grams), volume (cups/tablespoons and liters/milliliters, or where applicable the size or numbers of units), for example:

Strawberries, 5.5 oz (156 g), 1 cup (237 ml):   45 cal
Onions, chopped: 3 oz (85 g), $1/2$ cup (118 ml):   36 cal
Orange, 7 oz (199 g), 3" (7.6 cm) diameter: 60 cal
Almonds, whole, 1 oz (28.4 g), 24 individual almonds: 170 cal
   (Good luck measuring odd-shaped nuts in tablespoons like some books recommend!)

Your book should include meats, poultry, and fish listed by raw as well as cooked weight, and method of cooking (e.g., dry heat like baking or roasting versus moist heat like steaming or stewing). This is important because foods generally lose water as they cook, especially when cooked with dry heat—water loss makes the cooked food somewhat more calorie dense. Basically, if you take 4 ounces of raw lean meat, you can cook it any which way—dry roast it or steam it—and the calorie count won't change if the food loses or gains water (though at the risk of confusing you, I should point out that fattier cuts of meat may lose some fat as it renders out of the meat, and this loss of fat would obviously decrease the relative calories somewhat; but this should be irrelevant because these are the meats we ask you to avoid precisely because of their higher fat content).

Farmed Atlantic salmon, raw, 3 oz:	156 cal
Farmed Atlantic salmon, baked, 3 oz:	175 cal

Your book should also include a reference guide that clarifies whether the weight includes skin and bones. For example:

Chicken breast, edible weights (no bone):

Raw, w/skin, 5 oz:	240 cal
Raw, without skin, 4.5 oz:	130 cal
Roasted, w/ skin, 3.5 oz:	195 cal
Roasted, without skin, 3 oz:	140 cal

(Notice that 0.5 ounces of raw chicken skin accounts for 110 calories in the raw poultry, as opposed to 0.5 ounces of roasted skin only accounting for 55 calories—this is because much of the fat has rendered out during the cooking process, as was mentioned earlier.)

It also should include a section illustrating how to read food labels, as well as calorie and nutrition information for fast-food and sit-down restaurants. FYI, when food is prepared, the more food surface area exposed to oil, the more outrageous the calorie count:

½ medium baked potato (4 oz)	87 cal
Potato cut in half, fried (in oil)(4 oz)	207 cal
Fries, large cut (4 oz)	293 cal
Fries, skinny (4 oz)	353 cal
Potato chips (4 oz)	600 cal

(The preceding information is adapted from "*The Calorie King Calorie, Fat and Carbohydrate Counter*" by Allan Borushek, which fulfills most of the above requirements). Keep your food records by hand for optimal calorie-counting accuracy; you can later transfer your data to an Internet site such as www.calorieking.com, www.fitday.com, www.caloriesperhour.com, my-calorie-counter.com, or sparkpeople.com, which will detail not only your foods' calorie values but also their nutrient contents.

Calorie-Counting Questions:

Question: When should I weigh my food versus sizing it up in a measuring cup or spoon?
Answer: Use measuring cups/spoons for liquids, semi-liquids (like yogurt or mustard), and very small items that pour easily (like sesame seeds or dry couscous). You will get a more accurate calorie count by weighing most other foods. Obviously, it would be next to impossible to judge exactly how many walnuts fit into one tablespoon because their irregular shapes stick out over the top of the spoon. But 1 ounce of walnuts has the same number of calories, whether they're finely chopped or whole and irregularly shaped.

Question: Do I weigh my food cooked or uncooked?
Answer: There's no perfect system. If you're preparing your own food, it might be easier to calculate calories based on the raw weight (although for foods like raw chicken that may be contaminated with bacteria, it involves some extra dish- and hand-washing). Then, if you take added cooking oils and "grilled-out" fat into account, regardless of the cooking technique, whether it's hydrating or dehydrating, the caloric total of the food remains the same. But sometimes a food has already been cooked—it's perfectly reasonable to weigh it after cooking, too. The bottom line is, understand the above principles, then do whatever seems easiest to you.

Question: What if my food's weight is different from the weight listed in my reference book?

Answer: Grab a calculator and use this equation:

My food's weight (or volume) ÷ listed weight (or volume) x listed calories = my food's calories

Let's say I'm about to snack on an apple that weighs 7.2 ounces, and my reference book lists an 8-ounce apple for 110 calories. You know your apple is only 90 percent (7.2/8.0) of the weight of the reference apple, so multiple 0.9 x 110 calories = 99 calories for my apple. Alternatively, many online sources will allow you to enter the exact weight of your food and calculate your calories automatically.

Question: What if my kitchen scale only measures foods in pounds and ounces, but my reference (like the nutrition label on the package) only lists the food's weight in grams?

Answer: There are 454 grams per pound, 16 ounces per pound, and 28.4 grams per ounce, so

Divide grams by 28.4 to get ounces.

Multiply ounces by 28.4 to get grams.

Similarly on the volume front:

Divide milliliters by 237 to get cups (8 fl oz).

Multiply cups by 237 to get milliliters.

Portion Control

Study after study confirms that overweight people *underestimate* the number of calories they consume (and *overestimate* their exercise and activity). Some of this is based on our tendency to underestimate portion sizes. Pour a bowl of cereal. Is that a single serving? No, most Americans pour out three servings or more! Order a pasta dish at your favorite Italian restaurant. A single serving? No, you're being wooed by three to four servings; a single ½-cup, 100-calorie offering seems pretty puny on our 21st century 13-inch plates (in the old days a 9-inch plate sufficed).

The answer to portion size awareness is a kitchen scale (they cost as little as $10), a measuring cup, and measuring spoon set. "Hand equivalencies" are a good backup if no scale is available:

one fist = 1 cup = two servings of whole-wheat pasta or oatmeal;

1 thumb = 1 ounce = one serving of low-fat cheese;

one palm or one deck of cards = 3 ounces = a cooked serving size for meat.

Eventually you'll get to the point where experience will allow you to accurately estimate portion sizes.

For those of you who loathe the idea of looking up each individual food's caloric value, you can use estimates. While this is not as effective as knowing the true number of calories you're consuming, estimating is still a world better than not paying attention at all! Use the following ballpark figures if you simply can't fathom the alternative:

Fresh fruit (apple, orange, peach, banana. etc.,): medium sized = 80 calories

1 cup tropical fruit/melons = 80 calories

1 ½ cups of berries = 80 calories

Cooked nonstarchy vegetables: ½ cup = 20 calories

Cooked oatmeal, rice, pasta, beans, or starchy vegetables: ½ cup = 100 calories

Cooked fish/poultry/lean red meat: 3 ounces = 125 calories

Nonfat dairy serving:

Milk/yogurt/(soymilk): 1 cup = 100 calories

Ricotta or cottage cheese: cup = 100 calories

Hard (reduced-fat) cheese: 1 ounce = 80 calories

Hidden Calories

They're everywhere! It's not uncommon for a chef to melt a pat of butter on your entrée as it leaves the kitchen to be delivered to your table. Sauces, gravy, oils, and dressings are also frequently tucked inside "healthy" foods. And then there are soft drinks, alcoholic beverages, and calorie-packed coffee drinks (lattes, etc.), and smoothies. These extras can add up—and if you're not on the lookout, you'll never see them!

Don't forget that restaurants are in business to please you, not vice versa. Request your food be prepared without added sugar, butter, or oils. Just asking for your fish to be grilled isn't specific enough—they'll slather it with butter or oil to keep it from sticking to the grill (and to satisfy your fat-addicted taste buds)! Added salt might be a problem for some, but is probably okay for you now because you've become a regular exerciser! Ask your server to remove the breadbasket from your table so that you aren't tempted to dig in. Order a double portion of steamed vegetables in place of the mashed potatoes or French fries. If your meal arrives and portions look too big, ask for them to immediately box half of your meal so that you don't find yourself finishing off the entire plate just because it's in front of you.

Reading Labels

Here's a real-life situation: I'm walking down a grocery store aisle with a third grader who yanks down a box of "Berry-Berry Kix" that he's seen advertised on TV and throws it in the cart. Plastered on the front of the box is a giant spoonful of what appears to be a healthy mix of cereal, raspberries, and blueberries. But when I read the ingredients on the label, there's not a spec of fruit! Prevention Institute released a study in 2007 revealing that this was not an isolated case. Shockingly, of 37 heavily advertised child-oriented foods packaged to imply they were fruit-based, over half (including Yoplait Go-Gurt Strawberry Splash yogurt) contain zero fruit! Many of the rest are "fat-trap" fruit drinks formulated with excess sugar and minimal fruit nutrients. Deceptive and misleading food-naming practices will not stop until we learn to read labels as well as we can read traffic signs and refuse to purchase items that have little or no nutritive value, despite what names the manufacturers give them for marketing purposes.

The obesity highway has on and off ramps too—which one will you and your family choose?

How Do You Divvy Up Your Daily Calorie Allotment?

It might seem a little complicated at first, but the basic goal is for you to split your calories relatively evenly and to eat approximately five to six meals/snacks throughout the day. The easiest way to do this is to divide your calories by four—one fourth of your daily calories is the approximate calorie amount that you should have for each of your three major meals, and then the last fourth should be split into two or three snacks or post-workout anabolic shakes.

As an example, let's say you're an ex-jock woman volleyballer who is 10 years and three kids removed from your gymnasium glory, with jiggly hip and belt overhangs. Your RDEE is 1,650 calories a day; 1,650 calories multiplied by a 0.8 correction factor equals 1,320 calories per day minimum (1,650 x 0.8 = 1,320). The basic plan is to divide 1,320 by four, which allots you about 330 calories for breakfast, 330 calories for lunch, and 330 calories for dinner, with the remaining 330 calories to be split between two or three snacks or post-workout shakes. See Table 10.1 for some sample menus.

Table 10.1 Sample Daily Menus for Various Calorie Allotments

Sample Day Menu (1,000 calories)

Meal	Menu	Calories
Anabolic shake:	1 serving "strawberry cheesecake" shake	177 calories
Breakfast:	¼ cup liquid egg substitute	30 calories
	Olive oil (use a mist sprayer–1 second)	10 calories
	2 tablespoons salsa	15 calories
	1 large low-carb La Tortilla Factory-brand tortilla	80 calories
Lunch:	2 cups romaine lettuce	15 calories
	½ cup red bell pepper	15 calories
	½ cup celery	7 calories
	5 cherry tomatoes	15 calories
	1 ounce cooked skinless chicken breast	50 calories
	2 tablespoons light balsamic vinaigrette	45 calories
Anabolic shake:	1 serving "strawberry cheesecake" shake	177 calories
Dinner:	3 ounces grilled yellowfin tuna	110 calories
	Olive oil, mist sprayer (1 second)	10 calories
	1 cup steamed broccoli spears	30 calories
	½ cup cooked brown rice	108 calories
Snack:	1 cup plain nonfat yogurt	100 calories
	3 ounces fresh blueberries	48 calories
TOTAL:		1,042 calories

Table 10.1 Sample Daily Menus for Various Calorie Allotments

Sample Day Menu (1,250 calories)

Meal	Menu	Calories
Anabolic shake:	1 serving "strawberry cheesecake" shake	177 calories
Breakfast:	¼ cup liquid egg substitute	30 calories
	Olive oil, mist sprayer (1 second)	10 calories
	2 tablespoons salsa	15 calories
	1 large low-carb La Tortilla Factory-brand tortilla	80 calories
Lunch:	2 cups romaine lettuce	15 calories
	½ cup red bell pepper	15 calories
	1 cup celery	14 calories
	10 cherry tomatoes	30 calories
	3 ounces cooked skinless chicken breast	150 calories
	2 tablespoons light balsamic vinaigrette	45 calories
Anabolic shake:	1 serving "strawberry cheesecake" shake	177 calories
Dinner:	3 ounces grilled salmon	175 calories
	Olive oil, mist sprayer (1 second)	10 calories
	1 cup steamed broccoli spears	30 calories
	½ cup cooked brown rice	108 calories
Snack:	1 cup plain nonfat yogurt	100 calories
	1 cup fresh blueberries	83 calories
TOTAL:		1,264 calories

Table 10.1 Sample Daily Menus for Various Calorie Allotments

Sample Day Menu (1,500 calories)

Meal	Menu	Calories
Anabolic shake:	1 serving "strawberry cheesecake" shake	177 calories
Breakfast:	1/4 cup liquid egg substitute	30 calories
	Olive oil, mist sprayer (1 second)	10 calories
	3 tablespoons salsa	22 calories
	1 large low-carb La Tortilla Factory-brand tortilla	80 calories
Lunch:	2 cups romaine lettuce	15 calories
	1/2 cup red bell pepper	15 calories
	1 cup celery	14 calories
	10 cherry tomatoes	30 calories
	3 ounces cooked skinless chicken breast	150 calories
	2 tablespoons light balsamic vinaigrette	45 calories
	1 cup skim milk	90 calories
Anabolic shake:	1 serving "strawberry cheesecake" shake	177 calories
Dinner:	3 ounces grilled salmon	175 calories
	Olive oil, mist sprayer (1 second)	10 calories
	1 cup steamed broccoli spears	30 calories
	1/2 cup cooked brown rice	108 calories
Snack:	1 cup plain nonfat yogurt	100 calories
	1/2 cup Kashi GoLEAN cereal	70 calories
TOTAL:		1,518 calories

The WOW! ℞ Hunger-Beater Snacks

BREAKFAST BURRITO

Canola or olive-oil spray (1 second)
¼ cup egg whites (or egg substitute)
1 large La Tortilla Factory–brand low-carb tortilla
2 tablespoons salsa
0.5 oz (2 tablespoons) light shredded mozzarella cheese

Heat small pan over medium heat and spray with oil; cook egg
whites. Add to tortilla along with salsa and cheese; wrap; microwave
30 seconds to melt cheese.

Calories: 155
Fat: 5 grams
Protein: 18 grams
Carbohydrates: 22.6 grams
Fiber: 14.5 grams

YOGURT & KASHI

1 container carb-reduced yogurt
½ cup Kashi GoLEAN cereal

Calories: 150
Fat: 2 grams
Protein: 18.5 grams
Carbohydrates: 19 grams
Fiber: 6 grams

APPLES & CHEESE

1 medium apple (5.4 oz), sliced
1 oz light string cheese

Calories: 140
Fat: 2.8 grams
Protein: 7.4 grams
Carbohydrates: 21.8 grams
Fiber: 3.7 grams

TURKEY WRAP

1 large La Tortilla Factory-brand low-carb tortilla
2 oz turkey breast lunch meat
2 teaspoons mustard

Calories: 146
Fat: 4.2 grams
Protein: 18.1 grams
Carbohydrates: 22.2 grams
Fiber: 14.3 grams

EDAMAME

1 cup steamed edamame (measured in pods)
2 tablespoons soy sauce

Calories: 165
Fat: 4 grams
Protein: 18 grams
Carbohydrates: 14.4 grams
Fiber: 10.3 grams

EGG & FRUIT

1 large hard-boiled egg
1 ½ cup whole strawberries

Calories: 147
Fat: 5.9 grams
Protein: 7.7 grams
Carbohydrates: 17.2 grams
Fiber: 4.3 grams

YOGURT & BERRIES

1 container zero-fat Greek yogurt
1 cup blueberries

Calories: 162
Fat: 0 grams
Protein: 14.3 grams
Carbohydrates: 26.9 grams
Fiber: 3.5 grams

CARROTS & HUMMUS

15 baby carrots
3 tablespoons hummus

Calories: 123
Fat: 4.2 grams
Protein: 4.1 grams
Carbohydrates: 18.4 grams
Fiber: 5.2 grams

Anabolic Shake Recipes

Drink only within 30 minutes after exercise to protect and feed muscle.

STRAWBERRY CHEESECAKE SHAKE

MAKES TWO SERVINGS

⅓ cup nonfat ricotta cheese
1 cup lactose-free nonfat milk
1 cup fresh or frozen whole strawberries, no added sugar
4 low-fat vanilla wafers
1 tablespoon honey

Place all ingredients in the blender and blend thoroughly (add ice as desired for optimal temperature and consistency).

Calories: 177
Protein: 10 grams
Fat: 0.5 grams
Carbohydrates: 33 grams

BLACK FOREST SHAKE

MAKES TWO SERVINGS

⅓ cup nonfat ricotta cheese
1 cup lactose-free nonfat milk
1 cup fresh or frozen cherries, no added sugar
Chocolate milk powder (2 tablespoons Nesquik, or 1 tablespoon Ovaltine)

Place all ingredients in the blender and blend thoroughly (add ice as desired for optimal temperature and consistency).

Calories: 150
Protein: 11 grams
Fat: 0 grams
Carbohydrates: 28 grams

JUST PEACHY SHAKE

MAKES TWO SERVINGS

⅓ cup nonfat ricotta cheese
1 cup lactose-free nonfat milk
1 cup frozen peach slices, no added sugar
2 tablespoon frozen orange juice concentrate
1 tablespoon honey

Place all ingredients in the blender and blend thoroughly (add ice as desired for optimal temperature and consistency).

Calories: 167
Protein: 11 grams
Fat: 0 grams
Carbohydrates: 32 grams

TROPICAL TREAT SHAKE

MAKES TWO SERVINGS

⅓ cup nonfat ricotta cheese
1 cup lactose-free nonfat milk
½ cup frozen mango chunks, no added sugar
½ small banana
2 tablespoons frozen pineapple juice concentrate

Place all ingredients in the blender and blend thoroughly (add ice as desired for optimal temperature and consistency).

Calories: 147
Protein: 10 grams
Fat: 0 grams
Carbohydrates: 27 grams

PURPLE COW SHAKE

MAKES TWO SERVINGS

$1/_3$ cup nonfat ricotta cheese
1 cup lactose-free nonfat milk
$1/_2$ cup frozen blackberries, no added sugar
$1/_2$ small banana
2 tablespoons frozen grape-juice concentrate

Place all ingredients in the blender and blend thoroughly (add ice as desired for optimal temperature and consistency).

Calories: 163
Protein: 11 grams
Fat: 0 grams
Carbohydrates: 30 grams

RASPBERRY LEMONADE SHAKE

MAKES TWO SERVINGS

$1/_3$ cup nonfat ricotta cheese
1 cup lactose-free nonfat milk
$1 1/_2$ cups frozen raspberries, no added sugar
2 tablespoons frozen raspberry-lemonade concentrate
1 tablespoon honey

Place all ingredients in the blender and blend thoroughly (add ice as desired for optimal temperature and consistency).

Calories: 185
Protein: 11 grams
Fat: 0.5 grams
Carbohydrates: 35 grams

BLUEBERRY-BANANA SHAKE

MAKES TWO SERVINGS

⅓ cup nonfat ricotta cheese
1 cup lactose-free nonfat milk
½ cup frozen blueberries, no added sugar
½ small banana
2 tablespoons frozen grape juice concentrate
1 tablespoon honey

Place all ingredients in the blender and blend thoroughly (add ice as desired for optimal temperature and consistency).

Calories: 196
Protein: 11 grams
Fat: 0 grams
Carbohydrates: 37 grams

CORE NUTRITION FACTS

Protein

The WOW! ℞ encourages roughly a 30 percent protein intake for the following reasons:

- Appetite suppression (you don't need to avoid carbohydrates to get this beneficial effect of protein)
- Facilitation of fat loss
- Greater retention of lean tissue
- Less decline in resting metabolic rate

Some doctors have been concerned that large protein intakes could adversely affect bone and kidney health long term. However, evidence suggests that when protein (especially dairy and plant protein) replaces highly refined "white" grains (bread, rice, cereals, and pasta), these potentially detrimental outcomes are mitigated by the relative abundance of micronutrients in the lean protein (such as calcium in milk or the potassium in legumes).

Carbohydrates

The WOW! ℞ aims for roughly 45 percent of your caloric intake to be carbs, mainly fruits, vegetables, and whole-wheat grains. As a rule, the typical American eats too many calories but too few fruits and vegetables. Forget vitamins, it's fruits and vegetables that work wonders: studies show they protect against hypertension, hypercholesterolemia, cardiovascular disease, osteoporosis, stroke, age-related memory and intellect declines, colorectal adenomas, benign prostatic hypertrophy, and probably several types of cancer. Obviously, in the long run, across-the-board low-carb diets are not healthy.

Fiber

Fiber is a "tree-bark" carbohydrate that the body can't absorb—therefore fiber has no calories. Fiber is, however, vital for health. It fills you up, thereby acting like a weight-loss potion. It slows the absorption of sugars and starches and blunts sugar swings, thereby acting like an anti-diabetic drug. It binds to bile acids, thereby lowering cholesterol absorption and lowering blood cholesterol by 5 percent or more. It prevents constipation, diverticulosis, and bowel cancers. It even lowers stroke risk.

High-fiber foods have 5 or more grams of fiber per serving; if you're an average American, you currently consume only 10 to 15 grams of fiber daily, half of the 25 to 30 grams that should be the goal amount for maximal health. On The WOW! ℞, you'll approach your goal amount of fiber if, each day, you eat the core foods listed previously, including ample fruits, vegetables, whole grains, nuts, and seeds. But increase your fiber intake gradually over a few weeks in order to minimize cramping, bloating, and rectal gas. This gives the helpful digestive bacteria in your gut—which can partially digest fiber and produce nonodorous gases as a by-product—time to adjust to your dietary fiber intake increase. (By the way, most odorous rectal gas results from the breakdown of fats and proteins.) Also, a high-fiber diet requires that you drink six-plus glasses of noncaloric fluids daily to ensure that the fiber doesn't sludge. Too much fiber (more than about 70 grams a day, which is possible in people who take handfuls of fiber supplements) may interfere with the absorption of trace minerals, including iron, zinc, magnesium, and calcium. Fortunately, this effect is minimal when you consume a high (25- to 30-gram) fiber diet, because high-fiber foods are rich in minerals.

Mercury

Elevated levels of mercury appear to attack the nervous system, contributing to behavioral problems and mild loss of intelligence in children. Studies also suggest exposure to elevated levels of mercury could adversely affect the immune and reproductive systems of adults. Recently, I've seen a number of well-to-do patients with unusually high mercury exposures; they subsist on fish because of taste preference and pursuit of health benefits. They think they're doing the right thing by regularly eating swordfish, sea bass, halibut, and ahi tuna steaks. Unfortunately, these species happen to have the highest content of mercury sold in restaurants and grocery stores.

I am a big believer in the health benefits of fish, but I counsel my patients to rely on low-mercury species such as wild salmon, sardines, sole, tilapia, or small shellfish. (Go online to *http://www.cfsan.fda.gov/~frf/sea-mehg.html* to view a comprehensive listing of high- and low-mercury species.) Limit sushi and tuna to one meal per week (canned light tuna is lower in mercury than albacore). Fertile women are advised to avoid moderate and high-mercury species altogether unless they are documented to have low baseline mercury levels.

Fats

For decades now, we've been bombarded with "fat is bad" warnings. But truth be told, not all fats are linked to disease—mono- and polyunsaturated fats (think fish with its omega-3 type of polyunsaturated fat and vegetable, tree nut, and avocado fat) in moderation appear to be "heart healthy." Evidence even suggests the much-maligned egg yolk may pack as much heart benefit (good fats lower bad cholesterol without interfering with the good-guy cholesterol) as risk (bad cholesterol) if eaten once a day. The problem with healthy fats? Calories! You have to eat less of something else—hopefully saturated (animal) fats or the refined and liquid carbs we as a country are drowning in. Surprisingly, eating more fat does not necessarily make your weight go up. Studies show either no relationship between fat intake and obesity, or in some cases a tendency for Europeans with the highest fat intake to be the thinnest. (With an understanding of the benefits of good fat, the blind effect of "fat-blocker" weight-loss pills becomes a little troubling.)

Still, overweight persons should eat only tiny quantities of good fats. A full avocado is somewhere north of 300 calories and can easily torpedo a 1,200-calorie diet; ditto for 18 cashews (165 calories), an injudicious tablespoon (3 teaspoons) of olive oil (120 calories), or a mere 3-tablespoon slab of natural peanut butter (300 calories).

Trans Fats

Trans fats are dangerous, worse even than saturated fats. They increase "bad" cholesterol (LDL), especially the small, dense LDL particles most damaging to arteries; they lower "good" cholesterol (HDL), amplify the tendency of blood platelets to clump into artery-blocking clots, and enhance inflammation, a covert activity of the immune system implicated in heart disease, stroke, and diabetes.

Food manufacturers initially embraced solid trans fats—created by bubbling hydrogen gas through relatively perishable liquid vegetable oils in the presence of a nickel catalyst—because it facilitated much longer shelf lives for prepared foods. Sizable quantities of this added fat were once found in essentially all store-bought cookies and other bakery products, crackers, and even frozen breakfast products.

However, as of January 1, 2006, trans fats must be listed on food labels along with other bad fats (saturated fats) and good ones (unsaturated fats). Now food companies are scrambling, and many have succeeded in going "trans fat free." Keep in mind, though, that according to the FDA, a product claiming to have zero trans fats can actually contain up to a half-gram (Canada set a different standard of zero as under 0.2 grams), so you still need to scan the ingredient list for "partially hydrogenated vegetable oil" and "vegetable shortening," especially if it's something you eat regularly. In some cases, trans fats have been replaced with old-fashioned saturated fats, so keep an eye on the total fat and saturated fat quantities on labels.

Nitrites and Nitrates

Nitrites and nitrates are used as food additives in cured and processed meats and some smoked fish. They give cured meats, like bacon and hot dogs, a pink color. Nitrates and nitrites also build up in the soil as a result of contamination with human sewage, animal manure, and nitro-

gen-based fertilizers. Infants are at risk when exposed to excessive levels of nitrates or nitrites because they can interact with other substances
in the body to form potential cancer-causing chemicals called *nitroamines.*
Although increased disease in adults has not been proven, it makes sense
to steer clear. Avoid processed meats; buy organic produce when possible (although there's no guarantee that "organic" produce has less pes-
ticide residues than copiously washed "regular" produce).

Food Freshness

When you purchase a prescription antibiotic at the local pharmacy, the
law requires an expiration date to appear on the packaging, indicating
when a sizable portion of that drug will have spontaneously degraded
into an inactive compound.

Isn't it wild how people will get crazed and throw out a recently expired antibiotic, but never give a thought about the freshness of their
food? Food freshness is more important! Why? An antibiotic expiration
date may indicate that about 10 percent of the original antibiotic is inactive—fortunately, inactive antibiotic compounds are not harmful, and
since the vast majority of an active drug still remains intact, if you pop
a recently "expired" antibiotic, you'd be none the worse for your frugal
ways. Not so for food! When food expires, not only are vital antioxidants
lost (meaning you're going to have to consume a lot more calories to get
the same amounts of micronutrients), but the "lost" antioxidants can
also flip, becoming "oxidants," miniscule pro-aging, pro-inflamma-
tory double agents.

Sure, if you're starving in a jail cell in Afghanistan, chained against
a concrete wall, you will eat a soft brown banana and a chicken leg that
smells funky. In that situation, you're subconsciously making a practical trade-off by consuming much-needed calories, protein and minerals despite the hit your body's self-defense system will take from eating
food-borne oxidants.

Understandably, all animals have a powerful aversion to rancid food. But how can we human beings know when food is fresh, and therefore contains the most advantageous amounts and ratios of antioxidants and other micronutrients? Become aware of expiration dates that are required on many foods, especially perishable items such as fish, poultry, meat, dairy products, and even eggs. Consume the freshest food that's available to you.

Fresh Fruit

Are you baffled when it comes to selecting high-quality fruit at the market? I know I was. In fact, I was beyond baffled; I was angry. As opposed to selecting prime fresh vegetables, which was a relative no-brainer, half the fruit my wife or I brought home tasted awful or, worse yet, was moldy by the time we got around to pulling it out of the fridge. That's when I decided to look into this fruit conundrum, partly because I was so mad, partly because as a doctor preaching fruit consumption, I was embarrassed by how little I knew.

We've all suffered through tart oranges, rubbery green bananas, concrete-hard pears, and juiceless apples, not to mention peaches either picked too early or not allowed to properly ripen. And we've all dumped fruit ripened past its prime, regrettably often after we've taken a wicked bite (recently a patient of mine in the strawberry business was bragging about his biggest customer—the garbage can!). Ideally, we'd go to a true local farmer's market each day and purchase perfectly ripe fresh fruit to eat that same day. Well, few of us have access to a daily farmer's market, and perhaps that's no great loss because I've heard rumors that some local farmer's market vendors—unless they happen to also be the growers—get their products from the same supplier as the grocery stores. If we can't purchase fruit directly from the growers, then going to the neighborhood supermarket every day is the way to go, right? Fat chance! Most Americans would subsist on Uncle Ben's instant rice and leftover Halloween candy before agreeing to drive in, appraise the produce, and stand in a checkout line every 24 hours—even with those great rag-sheet headlines to browse.

Can you procure perfect fresh fruit without living at the grocery store or becoming a professional dessert chef? Yes, but you need a cheat sheet.

The Tsama Melon: The World's Most Indispensable Fruit.

The entire San Bushman tribe, which ekes out a living on the Kalahari Desert days away from civilization, shockingly exists with zero water resources during the drought season. Their only source of liquid is the tsama melon (90-plus percent water by weight), which they religiously stockpile in the shade, protected from poaching wild animals inside a prickly fence. This tasty watermelon-like fruit is a veritable lifesaver. If you're ever lucky enough to tour Botswana, try one.

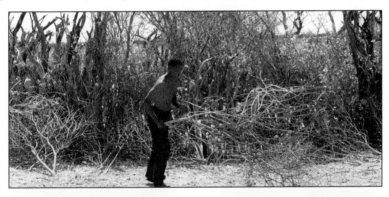

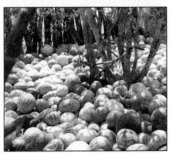
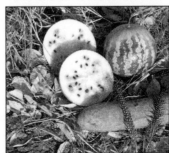

FRESH-FRUIT CHEAT SHEET

Use these guidelines when shopping and purchasing your weekly fruit:

- One shopping trip per week.
- Purchase three (different-colored) portions of fruit per day, per person, preferably one a high-vitamin-C variant (21 portions of fruit per person per week), according to this freshness formula:
  - Monday fruit: Ripe when it's picked; short shelf life; eat during the first few days.
  - Wednesday fruit: Ripe when it's picked; longer shelf life, eat midweek.
  - Friday fruit: Not ripe when picked; longest shelf life, eat at end of week or later.
- As a fallback option, have all varieties of frozen fruit stockpiled in your freezer—compared to prime fresh fruit, the taste may be down a notch or two, but the nutrient value is nearly identical (they're usually flash-frozen immediately after picking) and when purchased in bulk they're easier on the wallet.
- Bring a calculator to the fruit section. The prices are obviously meant to obfuscate the true price of each fruit. Rather than sell fruit by the pound, I was amazed to see berries variously sold in 4.4, 5.6, 11, 12, 15, and 16-ounce baskets, not to mention by pints and half-pints! And there's good reason to confuse the consumer. Some fruit goes for over 22 bucks a pound! Prices for the same quality fruit from store to store varied by as much as 300 percent! Sometimes frozen fruit was the exact same price as fresh (especially in cheaper fruits), but other times frozen cost only a fifth as much as fresh fruit!
- Interpret "antioxidant" potency studies with a grain of salt. Blueberries are bursting with anthocyanins, the substance that makes them—and subsequently your lips and teeth—a deep blue. A recent Tufts University study of 60 fruits and vegetables rated blue-

berries highest of all in antioxidant power. Soon after this study hit the local newspapers, I discovered some of my patients were eating only blueberries every day.

I don't think this is wise because our bodies co-evolved millions of years ago with a wide variety of fruits and vegetables containing a massive array—literally thousands—of unique antioxidants. Attempts to rate the pro-health "powers" of various foods is difficult because different research assays give conflicting results and no one is sure exactly how much of the "super-food's" vital ingredients are absorbed or whether the antioxidants in question need to be accompanied by other cofactors to be effective. Multiple studies suggest increased fruit and vegetable intake decreases disease; on the other hand, no single antioxidant has ever been shown to decrease disease. The color of fruits and vegetables— based on a unique spectrum of light-adsorbing phytonutrients— signals the type of antioxidant inside.

Given the above observations, it makes most sense to rotate through as many colors (red, purple, orange, yellow, green, dark green, and white) of vegetables and fruits as possible.

Buying Tips for Monday Fruit

For blackberries, blueberries, raspberries,* strawberries,* cherries, and grapes: (* denotes vitamin C–rich fruits.)

- Purchase seven portions of these delicate, ready-to-eat varieties (per person you're shopping for) for consumption early in the week.
- Monday fruit does not ripen after it's picked. Has it been picked too early? Will it never reach its full taste potential? Or was it plucked at just the right moment, stored and transported in a

timely fashion, and is now exploding with flavor? Sneak a taste, if possible! (Yes, some markets will even accommodate your request for a sample taste.)

- Berries are low in calories and high in fiber, but are some of the most delicate (and expensive at over $22 a pound!) fruits available. Inspect their container for dampness or stains, which may indicate that there are crushed, moldy, or decaying berries under the top layer.
- When you get home, remove fruit from their containers and throw away any mushy fruit—one rotten berry or cherry in a bin can set off a chain reaction of decay.
- Refrigerate unwashed on paper towels; set aside soft, overripe fruit to eat right away.
- Leave the leafy caps and stems intact until eating, because once the caps/stems are removed, the fruit can dehydrate—or absorb water during washing. Use scissors to cut off small clusters of grapes from the stem, instead of picking individual grapes off, to prevent drying.
- Rinse only before eating—washing removes a protective barrier and can also cause the fruit to absorb excess water.
- Monday fruit can turn mushy and moldy within two to three days—so consume early in week or flash-freeze for later use.

Buying Tips for Wednesday Fruit:

For apples, cantaloupe,* grapefruit,* oranges,* pineapples,* tangerines,* lemons, and watermelon:

- Purchase seven portions of these hearty, ready-to-eat varieties (per person you're shopping for) for consumption mid-week.
- Thick skin prevents decay and prolongs shelf life—grapefruits are especially hardy (please, never ruin the taste of this delicious

fruit by dumping on sugar!).

- Good-quality cantaloupes are pleasantly fragrant and often have a distinctive patch of bleached color (resulting from when the melon ripened on the vine, its weight resting on the hot soil). Similarly, a ripe watermelon will have a yellow underside (rather than greenish or white).
- Examine melon stem ends; they should be moist, not moldy, and have a slight indentation. If the stem is green, the melon was picked too soon; if the stem has fallen off, the melon might be overripe.
- Avoid melons with soft spots, dark bruises, and cracks. Tap on the melon with your flat hand. When the note is deep and thick, the melon is ripe and sweet.
- Consumers have a problem with pineapples: its ripeness is tough to judge.

The sweetness of fresh pineapple, like melons, results when starch stored in the stem of the plant converts to sugar, which then enters the fruit. Therefore, growers should allow pineapples to fully ripen on the plant, then harvest and ship as quickly as possible, because a pineapple will not get any better, only older.

A subprime, picked-too-soon-pineapple can still have golden yellow skin; thumping tests or pulling a leaf from its crown to see how loose it is will only tell you how old a pineapple is, not how sweet the fruit is inside.

The stem-smell test may be best, although if the pineapple is kept cold in the market, a fragrant aroma may not be apparent. In that case, put it in your grocery cart at the beginning of your shopping and conduct the sniff test after it's warmed up a bit (avoid if it smells sour or fermented).

The pineapple won't get any sweeter at home, but it will get a little softer and juicer if it's left at room temperature for a few days. If you store it upside down, the sweeter juice that has settled at the bottom will redistribute throughout the pineapple, making the taste more uniform.

- Wednesday fruit does not get sweeter after picked—but does "mature," getting softer/juicier if left at room temperature for several days. I prefer to then chill the fruit; however, be aware that some varieties may remain juicier if kept at room temperature (to thoroughly chill a large watermelon, plan on 12 hours of refrigeration).
- Even the inedible thick skins of Wednesday fruit should be washed just before eating—bacteria grow on their surfaces and can be transferred to the fruit inside during cutting.
- You can prevent cut apples from browning by rubbing the fruit with a mixture of lemon juice and water, or place peeled or sliced apples in cold water with a little lemon juice added.
- I realize Americans have a love affair with their morning orange juice. But please resist the juicing urge! Consume the whole fruit—get more filled up (same calories, way more fiber) and less of a sugar rush (the whole fruit has a lower glycemic index than the juice).

Buying Tips for Friday Fruit

For apricots, avocados, bananas, kiwi fruit,* mangos,* nectarines, peaches, papayas,* pears, plums, and pomegranates:

- Purchase seven portions of these not-yet-ready-to-eat varieties (per person you're shopping for) for consumption toward the end of the week or later.
- Matures after it's picked.
- Avoid fruit with signs of decay—bruised, shriveled, or mushy skin. Avoid rock-hard green fruit that was picked too soon and may never ripen with full flavor.
- Fresh pears, like bananas, are unique fruit that ripen best off the tree. If left on the tree too long, their delicate flesh gets "gritty"—

I know, because I have a Bartlett pear tree and we're always trying to figure out how much yellow we need to see before picking! Hint: If picked green with the first hint of yellow, they'll turn a delicious bright yellow when ripening off the tree.

- Allow Friday fruit to age gracefully in a kitchen bowl at room temperature, away from heat and direct sunlight. If you want this fruit to ripen more quickly, place together in a loosely closed brown paper bag (in the kitchen bowl). To further accelerate the process, add a nearly ripe banana or apple to the "ripening" bag.
- A rock-hard avocado will ripen at room temperature in about five days, faster if placed in a paper bag with a tomato.
- How do you tell when this fruit is ripe and ready to eat? Place the fruit in your palm and squeeze gently. If it gives just slightly, you're in business. Pears ripen from the inside out, so when their body is squishy, you're too late; instead, the proper gauge for a pear is if the stem area indents when you gently press there. When fruit passes the gentle squeeze or indent test, eat it immediately or refrigerate for another few days.
- Never refrigerate green bananas; cold temperatures interrupt the ripening process, which will not resume even when the fruit is returned to room temperature! Hard, green bananas have an astringent taste—they're safe to eat but are harder to digest than soft, sweet, creamy, ripe bananas.
- Rinse under cold running water just before you're ready to eat.
- Once cut and exposed to air, avocado flesh (like a fresh-cut potato or apple) oxidizes and turns dark within minutes. To keep the flesh fresh, rub on lemon or lime juice; add the juice to mashed avocado when making guacamole. Plastic wrap is needed to protect a halved avocado overnight in the refrigerator.

Table 10.2 Sample Fruit Values

Fruit	Calories	Vitamin C	Potassium	Folic Acid	Fiber
(One serving)		mg	mg	mcg	grams
		RDA	RDA	RDA	RDA
		90mg men	3500mg	400 mcg	25 grams
		75mg women			
Apple	81 (1 sm/6 oz)	7	165	4	4
Apricot	68 (4 med)	14	364	12	3
Avocado - California	73 (¼ med)	4	220	39	3
Avocado- Florida	92 (¼ med)	13	267	27	4
Banana	90 (1 sm/6")	9	386	9	2
Blueberries	81 (1 cup)	19	112	9	4
Cantaloupe	80 (1½ c diced)	86	626	49	1.5
Cherries	74 (1 cup sweet)	8	260	5	2.5
Grapefruit	88 (1 med)	78	338	28	1
Grapes	83 (¾ cup)	13	230	2	1
Kiwi fruit	92 (2 med)	141	474	38	4
Lemon	72 (3 med)	134	348	28	6
Mango	104 (½ med)	48	152	15	3
Nectarine	67 (1 med)	12	288	7	2
Orange	75 (1 sm/6 oz)	89	250	52	3
Papaya	74 (½ lg)	118	489	72	3.5
Peach	60 (1 lg/5.5 oz)	10	298	6	2
Pear	80 (1 sm/5 oz)	6	165	10	4
Pineapple	74 (1 cup)	56	178	23	2
Plum	73 (2 med)	21	227	6	2
Pomegranate	104 (1 med)	16	399	9	1
Raspberries	96 (1½ cups)	48	228	18	12
Strawberries	92 (2 cups)	169	440	69	6
Tangerine	74 (2 med)	45	278	26	3
Watermelon	70 (1½ cups)	19	260	7	1.5

Chapter Eleven

Mind Over Matter

THE WEIGHT, CALORIE, AND EXERCISE JOURNAL

"Journalers" lose significantly more fat than "nonjournalers." Make every attempt to journal for at least the first four months of The WOW! ℞. You won't regret it.

Table 11.1 Sample Weight, Calorie, and Exercise Journal

Name: Jane Smith		RDEE 1562	RDEE x 0.8 1250	WOW! Weight 158 lbs	
Date	Weight[a]	Calories	Aerobic vigorous[b]	Aerobic moderate[c]	Anaerobic/ aerobic PPT training[d]
	lbs	kcal/d	hrs/d	hrs/d	hrs/d
8/6-Mon	218	1255	1.5		0.5
8/7-Tues		1242	1	1.5	
8/8-Wed		1329	1	0.5	0.5
8/9-Thur	216	1255			
8/10-Fri		1221	1.5		0.5
8/11-Sat		1301		2.75	
8/12-Sun		1246	1	0.5	
8/13-Mon	213				

[a]weight to be taken first thing in AM in underwear
[b]vigorous = jogging at 5 mph or more intense
[c]moderate = exercise with intensity similar to walking
[d]PPT training should have few if any break periods
NOTE: Daily weights are optional, except for Monday mornings, which are mandatory.

THE FIVE-POINT WOW! ℞ THOUGHT JOURNAL

Keeping a thought journal may help you identify events, situations, or feelings that trigger overeating. It may also help you identify automatic or instant thoughts you experience that have detrimental effects on your behavior. Awareness is the first step to change!

1. When an emotional event occurs (this may be overeating or something that led to overeating), write down what happened.
2. Next, jot down two or three feelings you experienced in connection with the event, for example: I felt *sad, angry, irritated, drained, embarrassed, exhausted, scared, devastated, overwhelmed, anxious, frustrated, blue, nervous, hopeless, afraid, enraged, helpless, cheerful, ecstatic, excited, giddy, hopeful....*
3. After that, ask yourself what was going through your mind the instant you felt those emotions and write that down. These are the "automatic thoughts" that we experience from moment to moment—for example, "I always ruin everything!"
4. Evaluate whether you believe the automatic thought to be true or whether it's inaccurate. Many of our automatic thoughts are self-defeating and may fall into one of these categories:
   a. All-or-nothing thinking—looking at everything as black or white rather than shades of gray.
   b. Overgeneralization—applying one situation to your whole life, as a never-ending pattern.
   c. Catastrophization—perceiving an issue to be bigger than it is (making a mountain out of a mole hill).
   d. Mind reading—assuming that you know what others are thinking or saying about you.
   e. Fortunetelling—assuming that you know exactly what will happen next.
   f. Negative thinking—ignoring or failing to see positive things/traits.

g. Victim mentality—unrealistic belief that bad things happen only to you.

h. Labeling—calling yourself names, or reasoning based on a label rather than on a more complete picture.

5. If your automatic thought contained self-defeating thinking, write a revised response from a more balanced perspective—what you would tell a friend if you were counseling them about this problem.

Examples of the Five-Point WOW! ℞ Thought Journal in Action:

1. **The Event:** I ate three pieces of cheesecake after my boss criticized my work and asked me to revise it.
2. **Feelings:** Guilty, tired, defeated.
3. **Automatic Thoughts:** "My boss thinks I'm an idiot."
4. **True?** Probably not—if my boss thought I was an idiot, he/she would have fired me. My automatic thought fell under the "mind-reading" category—assuming I know what others are thinking about me.
5. **Revised Response:** "It was just constructive criticism, not a comment on me personally or my abilities."

1. **The Event:** My boyfriend broke up with me, so I pigged out on ice cream!
2. **Feelings:** Depressed, lonely, devastated.
3. **Automatic Thoughts:** "I'm a loser and no one will ever love me."
4. **True?** No—though my boyfriend doesn't think it will work out, he was attracted to me and other people will be, too. My automatic thoughts fell under the "labeling" and "fortune-

telling" categories—calling myself names and assuming I know what will happen in the future.

5. **Revised Response:** "Though this relationship wasn't meant to be, it is not because I am a loser. I might be sad now, and that's OK, but there will be other boyfriends in the future!"

---

1. **The Event:** I've been eating comfort food and haven't exercised for three days because I've been stressed out about my mother-in-law's visit.
2. **Feelings:** Anxious, irritated, drained.
3. **Automatic Thoughts:** "My weight-loss plan is ruined—I may as well give up because I'll never be able to lose the weight."
4. **True?** No. My automatic thoughts fell under the "all-or-nothing" and "catastrophization" categories—seeing the plan as black or white and assuming that a few days of being off the plan is the end of the world.
5. **Revised Response:** "Everyone has ups and downs, and just because I've been off the plan for a few days doesn't mean it's ruined forever or that I can't do it—I just need to get back on the wagon and keep at it."

ANXIETY AND DEPRESSION SCALE

Choose one response from the four given for each interview. Give an immediate response; don't think too long about your answer. The questions relating to anxiety are marked "A" and to depression "D." The score for each answer is given in the right column. Answer each question based on how you currently describe your feelings.

A–I feel tense or "wound up":

      Most of the time   3

      A lot of the time   2

      From time to time, occasionally   1

      Not at all   0

D–I still enjoy the things I used to enjoy:

      Definitely as much   0

      Not quite so much   1

      Only a little   2

      Hardly at all   3

A–I get a sort of frightened feeling, as if something awful is about to happen:

      Very definitely and quite badly   3

      Yes, but not too badly   2

      A little, but it doesn't worry me   1

      Not at all   0

D–I can laugh and see the funny side of things:

      As much as I always could   0

      Not quite so much now   1

      Definitely not so much now   2

      Not at all   3

A–Worrying thoughts go through my mind:

      A great deal of the time   3

      A lot of the time   2

      From time to time, but not too often 1

      Only occasionally   0

D–I feel cheerful:

Not at all	3
Not often	2
Sometimes	1
Most of the time	0

A–I can sit at ease and feel relaxed:

Definitely	0
Usually	1
Not often	2
Not at all	3

D–I feel as if I am slowed down:

Nearly all the time	3
Very often	2
Sometimes	1
Not at all	0

A–I get a sort of frightened feeling like "butterflies" in the stomach:

Not at all	0
Occasionally	1
Quite often	2
Very often	3

D–I have lost interest in my appearance:

Definitely	3
I don't take as much care as I should	2
I may not take quite as much care	1
I take just as much care as ever	0

A–I feel restless like I have to be on the move:

Very much indeed	3
Quite a lot	2
Not very much	1
Not at all	0

D–I look forward with enjoyment to things:

As much as I ever did	0
Rather less than I used to	1
Definitely less than I used to	2
Hardly at all	3

A–I get sudden feelings of panic:

Very often indeed	3
Quite often	2
Not very often	1
Not at all	0

D–I can enjoy a good book or radio or TV program:

Often	0
Sometimes	1
Not often	2
Very seldom	3

Scoring (Add the As = Anxiety. Add the Ds = Depression). The norms below will give you an idea of the level of anxiety and depression.

0–7 = Normal

8–10 = Borderline abnormal

11–21 = Abnormal

Reference: Zigmond AS, Snaith RP. Acta Psychiatr Scand. 1983 Jun;67(6):361-70

APPENDIX

The Biggest Loser Pre-participation Medical History Form

Name: _____

Occupation: _____ Date: _____

Married/single: _____ Age of children: _____

Weight: _____ Weight one year ago: _____ Weight age 21: _____

Sizes? Pants (waist [in]): _____ Dress or shirt (collar) size: _____

Current medical problems (please list with name of treating health professional):

1.

2.

3.

Specifically, do you currently have symptoms of:

4. Esophageal reflux: heartburn, back of the throat sour taste or throat clearing? Yes/No

5. Wheezing, chronic cough, inappropriate shortness of breath (asthma)? Yes/No

6. Snoring, daytime tiredness, almost falling asleep while driving or at work? Yes/No

7. Episodes of upper-right abdominal pain? Yes/No

8. Hair loss? Yes/No

9. Depression, anxiety, food bingeing, or anorexia/bulimia? Yes/No

10. During exercise, have you felt dizzy, passed out, had chest or neck pressure, wheezing, cramping, dehydration, or overheating (heat exhaustion)? Yes/No

11. Has a health professional ever told you (circle appropriate entries):

    a. You're diabetic or prediabetic? Yes/No

    b. You have high blood pressure? Yes/No

    c. You have gallstones or kidney stones? Yes/No

    d. You have high cholesterol? Yes/No

e. You have high uric acid or gout? Yes/No

f. You have sleep apnea? Yes/No

g. You are overweight/obese/morbidly obese? Yes/No

h. You have a bleeding disorder, thyroid disease, heart disease, arthritis, cancer, seizures, a psychiatric disorder, or sickle cell trait? (circle)

12. Have you ever been told you have any other type of disease?

_____

13. List hospitalizations/surgeries:

    1.

    2.

14. Has a health professional ever recommended weight-loss surgery? Yes/No

15. Please list all current prescription and over-the-counter medications (include vitamins, antacids, and appetite suppressants).

    1.

    2.

    3.

16. Allergies to medications (list with type of reaction[s])?

    1.

    2.

17. Food allergies or intolerances (i.e., lactose intolerance)?

18. Were your routine childhood vaccinations given? Yes/No

19. Cigarette use per day? _____

20. Alcohol use per day? _____

21. Recreational or street drug use, including marijuana? (past treatment?) _____

22. Are you on a special diet now? Yes/No. If so, what type?

_____

23. When was your last "weight-loss" diet?

24. During your last "weight-loss" diet, how much weight did you lose? _____

25. Your current exercise—types, durations, intensity—average over the last two months:
    a. Vigorous aerobic exercise (jogging intensity or greater) hrs/wk _____
    b. Moderate aerobic exercise (walking intensity) hrs/wk

    _____

    c. Weightlifting hrs/wk _____
26. Do you require orthotics or any braces? Yes/No? If so, specify _____
27. Number of years you played JV or varsity high school sports?

    _____

28. Current orthopedic problems limiting exercise? Yes/No? If yes: _____
29. Past orthopedic problems:
    a. Joint arthritis or pain? (Specify: feet, ankles, knees, hips, lower back, neck, shoulders, elbows, hands.)
    b. Muscle pulls. Yes/No.   If so, specify _____
    c. Tendonitis. Yes/No.   If so, specify_____
    d. Bursitis. Yes/No.   If so, specify_____
30. Family History: Do any of your siblings, aunts, uncles or either of your parents have:
    a. Obesity? Yes/No
    b. High blood pressure? Yes/No
    c. High cholesterol? Yes/No
    d. Gout? Yes/No
    e. Kidney stones or gallstones? Yes/No
    f. Diabetes? Yes/No
    g. Heart disease? Yes/No
    h. Sudden death? Yes/No
    i. Sickle cell anemia? Yes/No
    j. Easy bleeding? Yes/No
    k. Weight-loss surgery? Yes/No

31. Your Schedule:

    a. Do you eat at the same times each day? Yes/No

    b. Do you work out at the same time each day? Yes/No

    c. Do you go to bed at the same time each day? Yes/No

    d. Do you get up at the same time each day? Yes/No

    e. How many times do you weigh yourself per week? _____

    f. Number of hours per day you now watch TV? _____

    Home computer? _____

32. Self Evaluation:

    a. Energy Score (10–brimming with vigor; 1–tired, listless all the time)

    10 9 8 7 6 5 4 3 2 1

    b. Depression Score (10–down most days, low motivation; 1–optimistic, outgoing)

    10 9 8 7 6 5 4 3 2 1

    c. Relationship Score (10–great companionship and intimate relations; 1–impending split)

    10 9 8 7 6 5 4 3 2 1

    d. Overall Quality of Life (10–extremely pleased with all aspects of life; 1–extremely frustrated, disappointed, or upset with my current life!)

    10 9 8 7 6 5 4 3 2 1

PERSONAL PHYSICIAN STATEMENT

I have examined _____ on
_____ (date).

There are/are not any limitations on his/her participation in a six-month moderately restricted caloric diet (80 percent of the calculated resting daily energy expenditure typically 1,100 to 1,500 kcal/d (obese women), 1,400 to 1,900 kcal/d (obese men).

There are/are not any limitations on his/her participation in a mixture of vigorous and moderate physical activity of 1,000–3,000 kcal/d.

Other remarks regarding the applicant's health:

_____

Physician name (printed)

_____

Physician signature _____
Physician telephone number _____

MEDICAL ARTICLES WRITTEN ABOUT *THE BIGGEST LOSER* CONTESTANTS

This first paper summarizes the eye-opening fat loss and almost miraculous disease "curing" I witnessed in the initial season of *The Biggest Loser*. Believe me—I had to pinch myself as I stared at the dramatic data from this small group. Had I backed into something huge? If in fact obesity was responsible for 300,000 to 400,000 excess deaths each year in this country alone—not to mention $100 billion in excess health care costs—maybe even an expensive, several-month boot camp like we built for *The Biggest Loser* contestants was well worth the time and money for regular obese folks.

However, I knew, more than cost and convenience, it was the medical and orthopedic problems, though transient and nonlimiting, that narrowed the appeal of this intense exercise-based approach to the general population. The question was: Would less-aggressive exercise with less supervision be safer and still work the same magic?

Dramatic Weight Loss, Hyperhydration, and Acute Myogenic Hyperuricemia with Four-Hours-per-Day Exercise and Moderate Caloric Restriction in Motivated Obese Subjects

Original Contribution, 2004

Robert Huizenga, M.D. and James Mirocha, Ph.D.(c)

ABSTRACT

Background: "Experts" recommended against strenuous exercise in sedentary obese individuals despite a lack of data on the amount of exercise that can safely be prescribed for unfit, obese individuals as an adjunct to moderate caloric restriction for optimal weight loss and cardiac risk-factor reduction.

Objective: To evaluate the safety and efficacy of four-hour-a-day exercise and calorie-restricted diets.

Design, Setting, and Participants: An observational study of unfit obese (body mass index 38.7 ± 8.5 Kg/m^2) adults aged 30.5 ± 6.0 years with multiple cardiac risk factors. Intervention: 12 subjects motivated by a chance to remain on a reality TV show were encouraged to exercise twice-a-day (for on average four hours per day, including one to two hours of vigorous exercise) and moderately calorie restrict (resting daily energy expenditure (RDEE) x 0.8) on a high-protein, low-fat diet for 22 weeks.

Results: Subjects lost 25.0±8.3% (p <.001) of their weight and 78.5±26.7% (p <.001) of their excess fat. Total fat loss/total weight loss was 84.6±17.7%. At day 7, marked changes in uric acid (102±31.3%), CPK (611±577%), and CO_2 (-19.0±12.0%) (p <.001) were noted. Significant hemodilution was seen with day 15 and day 24 plasma volumes increased 23.9±9.0% and 26.0±6.2% (p <.001) in the face of low urine sodiums and fractional excretion of sodiums. Over the 22-week course of the show, subjects reported multiple transient (7/12) and nonlimiting persistent (2/12) orthopedic complaints and mild hair loss (6/11); subjects also reported symptomatic resolution of reflux (5/5), asthma (3/4), anxiety (1/2), bulimia (1/1) and snoring (7/7 better or gone). Resolution of systolic (5/7) and diastolic HTN (6/7), abnormal CRP (3/3), elevated fasting insulin (2/2), hypertriglyceridemia (5/5), LDL cholesterol (8/9), and the metabolic syndrome (5/5) was documented. 3/3 subjects quit cigarettes. Weights 43 weeks post-show completion were stable (+2.0±8.5%, p >0.40).

Limitations: Small sample size, nonrandomized observational study.

Conclusions: Four-hour-a-day exercise and a moderately restricted diet in sedentary obese individuals resulted in dramatic weight loss, fewer health complaints, and marked improvements in CAD risk factors. Asymptomatic acute myogenic hyperuricemia and acidosis as well as orthopedic injuries and hair loss were also noted. Hyperhydration, dehydration and probable muscle hypertrophy complicated the interpretation of weight changes.

——— ——

Over the subsequent summer and fall, I was energized to see the following results come in to my laboratory that partially answered this question! First off, the amazing exercise capacity of every single obese participant suggested the initial observations from the 12 *Biggest Loser-1* contestants were generalizable to a much larger group. Secondly, sizable fat loss and presumed muscle gain data from 48 *Biggest Loser-2* (the *Special Home Edition*) participants with only 10 days of boot-camp training, and substantially less exercise and trainer supervision at home suggested less exercise with less supervision could be safer and still work magic!!! The next step: Somehow fund a comparison study of the now-standard *Biggest Loser* exercise and diet boot camp to an entirely home based program. . .

Two-A-Day Exercise and Moderate Caloric Restriction: A Novel Weight Loss Potion

Robert Huizenga, M.D. and James Mirocha, Ph.D.(c)

ABSTRACT

Background: The addition of mild physical exertion to a weight-loss diet appears only minimally superior to diet alone; experts have recommended against strenuous exercise in sedentary obese individuals.

Objective: To evaluate the effect of inpatient exercise and diet boot camp (BC) duration on weight loss, health habits, and CAD reduction in sedentary obese individuals.

Methods: Eighty-five sedentary obese (37.8 ± 6.7 Kg/m^2) individuals 31.1 ± 8.8 years old were observed. Sixty-four participated as TV contestants in BC for 10 days followed by:

Biggest Loser-1 - 5 extra weeks BC, then 15 weeks unsupervised at home (n=12)

Biggest Loser-2 - 6 extra weeks BC, then 28 weeks at home (n=14)

Biggest Loser-2 (Special Home Edition) - 19 weeks at home (n=38).

Twenty-one alternatives got "usual care" (UC) with no exercise or diet instruction.

Results: Total weight loss and total fat loss/total weight loss for *Bl-1, BL-2, BL-2 (SHE)* and UC respectively was $25.0 \pm 8.3\%$, $34.6 \pm 12.2\%$, $21.2 \pm 7.4\%$ and $1.3 \pm 5.9\%$ (p<0.001) and $84.6 \pm 17.7\%$, $98.9 \pm 19.9\%$, $101.1 \pm 20.3\%$ and unknown. Total weight loss for *BL-1* was $22.7 \pm 11.3\%$ (p > 0.49) one year after show completion. Exercise increased 13.5 ± 7.7 and 1.0 ± 2.0 hrs/wk while TV viewing decreased 11.5 ± 9.3 and 5.0 ± 5.5 hrs/wk for contestants and UC respectively (p<0.001). Resolution of heartburn, snoring, wheezing, systolic and diastolic hypertension, abnormal glucose or insulin levels, elevated LDL and CRP levels was seen in all contestants (p<0.01). Twenty-four medical and 13 orthopedic complications necessitated temporary withdrawal of contestants from show participation. Medical and orthopedic side effects were less common in *BL-2 (SHE)* compared to *BL-1* and *BL-2*.

Conclusions: Some sedentary obese and morbidly obese adults are capable of intense two-a-day exercise while restricting calories. Significant reductions occurred in weight, TV viewing, and CAD risk factors. Total fat loss ÷ total weight loss approached 1 consistent with muscle gain. Even minimal boot-camp stays followed by two-a-day exercise and moderate caloric restriction at home resulted in significant fat loss.

———— ————

It was apparent that for me to win over dubious medical editors and academic reviewers, I needed more sophisticated research equipment. I secured the state-of-the-art GE iDXA body-composition machine to corroborate my Bod Pod fat % results and an adjusted Xitron Hydra body water device (BIS) to validate my blood tests and prove indeed that muscle gains (not excess fluid) were responsible for lean tissue changes. But none of these technologies had been well tested in a morbidly obese population. First up, were these tests reproducible (see below)? Next, would iDXA (based on weak X-rays) match independently obtained Bod Pod (based on density measurements) and adjusted BIS (based on impedance to a spectrum of weak electrical currents) results (see www.the-wowrx.com)?

Precision of Lunar iDXA Total Body BMD and Composition Measurements on Obese Subjects

R Huizenga[1], MK Oates[2]

[1]Cedars Sinai Medical Center, Los Angeles, CA; [2]Santa Maria, CA

ABSTRACT

Dual-energy X-ray absorptiometry (DXA), the method of choice for measuring bone mineral density, is increasingly accepted as an accurate and convenient method for measuring regional and total body composition. The ongoing worldwide epidemic of obesity has heightened interest in body composition and its association with diseases related to obesity, particularly cardiovascular disease and type-2 diabetes. The ability to monitor change in body composition depends on the precision error of the measurement. Few studies have reported precision errors in obese subjects.

We used the Lunar iDXA (GE Healthcare) to determine total body precision in 29 obese participants (15 females and 14 males) in a televised weight-loss and exercise program. Each subject was measured twice with repositioning at the beginning of the weight-loss program. Precision was determined using the root-mean squared method. Subjects average (SD, range) age (33.4 yrs (7.5, 22.1-53.9)), height (173.2 cm (10.9, 157.5-193.8)), weight (128.8 kg (27.5, 91.8-181.4)), BMI (42.5 (4.9, 33.7-51.5)), and total % fat (42.5 [33.7-

51.5]) were reported. Precision errors (% CV) on these obese subjects were about 1% for total body % fat, BMC, and BMD, and about 1.5% for total body fat and lean mass. We conclude that Lunar iDXA precision on obese subjects was excellent.

Measurement	Mean	SD	% CV
BMC (g)	3342.7	37.05	1.1%
BMD(g/cm2)	1.373	0.017	1.2%
Fat (kg)	59.1	0.84	1.4%
Lean (kg)	67.6	1.01	1.5%
% Fat	47.2%	0.42%	0.9%

Finally, the most meaningful experiment ever conducted on national TV was complete! In both the two-month and eight-month (www.the-wowrx.com) study of unfit, predominantly morbidly obese participants, a three-day weight-loss seminar recommending two to two-and-a-half hours of exercise and moderate caloric restriction with weekly newsletters was as predictive of dramatic fat loss as live-in boot camps with daily trainer supervising four hours of exercise per day, TV filming, and large monetary inducements. *So two hours of exercise with no trainer supervision was indeed safer and still worked fat-loss and muscle-gain magic.*

Impact of Live-In Boot Camp, Exercise Duration, TV Filming, and Financial Incentives on Weight Loss in Obese Individuals

Robert Huizenga, M.D. and James Mirocha, Ph.D.(c)

ABSTRACT

Background: Reality weight-loss shows have documented dramatic results. How much of this weight loss is attributable to boot camps with high-duration exercise, ever-present trainers, TV filming, and cash prizes?

Methods: Sixty-two unfit participants (289±60 pounds, body mass index 43.3 ± 5.6) were studied:

1) in a filmed live-in "boot camp" with trainers monitoring four-hours-a-day exercise, moderate caloric restriction with a 1 in 14 chance to win a $250,000 prize (BC) (n=14).

2) resuming regular home lives while self-monitoring two-and-a-half hours-a-day exercise and moderate caloric restriction taught at a three-day seminar but no TV filming, no trainers, and a 1 in 36 chance to return mid-season to the filmed boot camp for a 1 in 8 shot at the $250,000 (a 1/288 chance to win prize) (H) (n=36).

3) resuming regular home lives with no diet or exercise instructions, no filming, no trainers, and no financial inducements (C) (n=12).

Results: Total exercise for BC, H and C women and men respectively was 3.8±1.7 and 5.9±1.2; 2.2±0.7 and 2.7±1.0; and 0.7±0.7 and 0.2±0.3 hours per day. BC, H and C women and men respectively consumed 69±7.9 and 62±7.0%; 70±5.7 and 70±9.7%; and unknown of their resting daily energy expenditure (RDEE). The total weight loss % at two months for BC, H, and C women and men respectively was 15.2 ± 4.1 and 17.5±3.8%; 12.3±4.3 and 14.9±4.6%; 0.7±4.3 and -0.4±2.9%. Both female and male BC and H participants lost significantly more weight than controls (p = 0.002); BC weight loss was not significantly different from H (females p = 0.10, males p=0.14).

Conclusions: In this two-month study of unfit, predominantly morbidly obese participants, a three-day weight-loss seminar recommending two-and-a-half hours of exercise and moderate caloric intake was as predictive of dramatic fat loss as live-in boot camps with daily trainer supervising four hours of exercise per day, TV filming, and large monetary inducements.

This study illustrated the importance of relative waist versus butt-fat deposition: marbled visceral organ fat in the waist region appeared to be a unique predictor of the metabolic syndrome (and therefore early death) in this group of obese subjects. The WOW! R̥ can very successfully reverse this syndrome, liposuction and diet-only plans are far less likely to be effective.

Body Composition with iDXA in Obese Subject with and without Metabolic Syndrome

MK Oates1, R Huizenga₂

₁Santa Maria, CA, ₂Cedars Sinai Medical Center, Los Angeles, CA

ABSTRACT

Obesity has a major impact on public health and health-related expenses. Increased fat mass and its regional distribution, especially in the abdomen, are important predictors of the risk of cardiovascular disease and type-2 diabetes, diseases prevalent in individuals with a complex of metabolic risk factors referred to as the metabolic syndrome.

Recently, 49 obese subjects (27 females, 22 males) took part in a televised weight-loss and exercise program. The average weight (SD, range) at baseline was 129.1 (27.1, 88.9-185.9) kg and average (SD, range) of BMI was 41.7 (5.2, 31-54.9). In addition to weight, a number of metabolic variables (fasting glucose, triglycerides, high-density lipoproteins (HDL)), blood pressure, waist circumference, and body-composition variables (android % f at, gynoid % fat, android gynoid % fat ratio, and total % body fat) measured by DXA (iDXA, GE Healthcare) were recorded.

Subjects with risk factors indicating metabolic syndrome (n = 31) were found to have significantly greater weight, BMI, waist circumference, A/G ratio (abdomen/hip % fat), TB fat, and TB lean than subjects (n = 18) without metabolic syndrome. There was no significant difference in total body % fat between subjects with and without metabolic syndrome, indicating that regional fat distribution is the more important indicator.

We conclude that regional DXA fat measurements, including the android/gynoid ratio, are significant predictors of subjects with metabolic syndrome in this population of obese subjects.

Metabolic Syndrome	Weight	BMI	Waist Circ	Android	Gynoid	A/G	TB Fat	TB Fat
	kg		cm	% Fat	% Fat	% Fat Ratio	%	g
Yes n=31	138.0	43.1	139.7	61.6%	50.6%	1.24	45.1%	61893
No n=18	114.0	39.3	129.4	62.5%	57.9%	1.09	48.8%	55293
P Value	0.0006	0.006	0.001	ns	0.0007	0.0004	ns	0.034

The Holy Grail: Evaluation of at-home as well as boot-camp participants revealed muscle (www.thewowrx.com) and often even bone gain (see below) in the face of dramatic fat loss. Weight loss under these conditions significantly increases one's chances of long-term fat-loss maintenance.

Effect of Dramatic Weight Loss on Regional and Total Body BMD of Obese and Morbidly Obese Subjects

HS Barden[1], MK Oates[2], R Huizenga[3].

[1]GE Healthcare, Madison WI, [2]Santa Maria, CA, [3]Cedars Sinai Medical Center, Los Angeles, CA

ABSTRACT

The effect of dramatic weight loss on bone densitometry measurements has never been studied. Researchers have shown significant dual-energy x-ray absorptiometry (DXA) bone mineral density (BMD) decrease in overweight individuals at fracture-relevant sites after 12 months with diet induced but not exercise induced ~10% weight loss.(Arch Intern Med 2006; 166:2502-10) However, researchers have suggested that DXA measurement of bone mineral content (BMC) or bone area in obese and morbidly obese subjects might be unreliable due to the negative effects of increased soft-tissue thickness and increased X-ray attenuation on bone-edge detection; Lunar iDXA (GE Healthcare) uses a high-definition detector to provide improved image quality, precision and accuracy, especially under these conditions.

Recently, we measured total body, lumbar spine (L1-L4) and proximal femur on 25 female (11 obese (BMI >30), 14 morbidly obese (BMI >40)) and 22 male (all morbidly obese) subjects at the beginning and end of an eight-month aggressive weight-bearing exercise and moderate caloric restriction program. Average (SD) weights at baseline were 110 kg (9.7 kg) and 152 kg (20.0 kg) for females and males, respectively. Average (SD) weight losses were 27.5 kg (12.1 kg) and 49.3 kg (20.0 kg) for females and males, respectively. Percent weight losses for females and males were ~25% and 32%, respectively.

BMD change with weight loss was minimal (-1% or less) for total body and total femur. Lumbar spine BMD increased 1.5% and 6% for females and males, respectively. Average changes in bone areas were negligible (<0.4%) for all regions, indicating consistent edge detection with changing body weight and no magnification errors due to changes in distance of the bone above tabletop. Regressions of BMD and area change with weight loss were nonsignificant for total body and total femur. There was a significant increase in BMD with weight loss in men at the spine. It is unclear if the larger increase in spine BMD seen in men versus women, despite losing a greater percent of their total weight, is related to observed greater weight-bearing aerobic and weightlifting exercise, greater initial percentage lean mass or hormonal differences.

We conclude that bone results with the iDXA appeared relatively unaffected by dramatic weight loss in these mostly morbidly obese subjects. BMD changes were minimal for all regions with the exception of L1-L4 in men, and bone area changes for all regions were negligible.

Table 11.2 Bone Densitometry Changes with Weight Changes in Obese Subjects

		Females	Males
		% Change (SD)	% Change (SD)
Total Body	BMD	-0.4% (1.5%)	-0.8% (2.6%)
	BMC	-0.7% (1.8%)	-1.0% (2.3%)
	Area	-0.3% (1.9%)	-0.1% (1.9%)
Spine L1-L4	BMD	1.5% (3.0%)	6.4% (4.2%)
	BMC	1.2% (4.1%)	6.3% (5.2%)
	Area	-0.3% (1.6%)	-0.2% (2.6%)
Total Femur	BMD	-1.1% (2.4%)	-0.4% (3.3%)
	BMC	-1.2% (2.7%)	-0.2% (3.7%)
	Area	-0.1% (1.5%)	0.2% (1.7%)

Stay abreast of the latest research results at www.thewowrx.com

BIO

Team doctor for the Los Angeles Raiders football team from 1983 to 1990, Dr. Huizenga chronicled his experiences in the book, *You're OK, It's Just a Bruise-A Doctor's Sideline Secrets about Pro-Football's Most Outrageous Team.* During its release in 1994, the controversial book sparked a national debate about steroid use and ergogenic aid in professional sports. The book ultimately served as the inspiration for the Oliver Stone film, *Any Given Sunday.*

A graduate of Harvard Medical School, Dr. Huizenga has been Chief Resident at Cedars Sinai Medical Center in Los Angeles and is currently Associate Professor of Clinical Medicine at UCLA. He is also in private practice in Beverly Hills, California. He has appeared as a health expert on many network news and interview shows and has testified as a medical expert in a number of high-profile trials. In addition to *The Biggest Loser,* his television and movie consulting credits include *Extreme Makeover, WorkOut, Student Body* and *Into the Wild.*

Index